The South Texas Health Status Review

Amelie G. Ramirez • Ian M. Thompson
Leonel Vela

Editors

The South Texas Health Status Review

A Health Disparities Roadmap

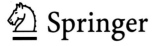 Springer

Editors
Amelie G. Ramirez
Institute for Health Promotion Research
University of Texas
Health Science Center at San Antonio
San Antonio, TX, USA

Ian M. Thompson
Department of Urology
UT Health Science Center at San Antonio
Cancer Therapy and Research Center
San Antonio, TX, USA

Leonel Vela
Regional Academic Health Center
UT Health Science Center at San Antonio
Harlingen, TX, USA

ISBN 978-3-319-00232-3   ISBN 978-3-319-00233-0 (eBook)
DOI 10.1007/978-3-319-00233-0
Springer Cham Heidelberg New York Dordrecht London

Library of Congress Control Number: 2013936723

Printed on acid-free paper

Springer is part of Springer Science+Business Media (www.springer.com)

Preface

South Texas is home to 18 % of the state's entire population.

That's 4.5 million people—an amount that could fill the home stadium of the NBA's San Antonio Spurs a whopping 242 times.

Yet South Texas residents, who are predominantly Hispanic/Latino, struggle with lower educational levels, less income, and less access to health care. This puts them in greater danger of facing dire health problems such as obesity or cancer.

The second edition of the *South Texas Health Status Review* is a comprehensive study of more than 35 health conditions and risk factors and how people in South Texas may be differently affected than those in the rest of Texas or the nation.

Does South Texas have higher breast cancer rates than the rest of Texas?

Do Hispanics in South Texas have more or less diabetes or obesity than Hispanics in the rest of the state?

This *Review* answers these and many other questions by: introducing each of the health conditions or risk factors; analyzing each condition or factor by age, sex, race/ethnicity, rural/urban location; and comparing the results between South Texas, the rest of Texas, and the nation.

The *Review*, originally published in 2008 and now updated in 2013, is a collaboration of the Institute for Health Promotion Research (IHPR) in the School of Medicine at The UT Health Science Center at San Antonio; the Cancer Therapy and Research Center (CTRC), a National Cancer Institute-designated Cancer Center at The UT Health Science Center at San Antonio; the Regional Academic Health Center (RAHC) at The UT Health Science Center at San Antonio; and the Texas Department of State Health Services.

We hope this *Review* gives researchers insight into inequalities that exist in South Texas—information that could stimulate and shape research and interventions to reduce or eliminate those very inequalities and improve the health of this large, diverse, culturally rich population.

Find the *Review* online at http://ihpr.uthscsa.edu.

Cite the *Review*:

Ramirez, A.G., Thompson Jr., I.M., and Vela, L. (Eds.). 2013. *The South Texas health status review: A Health Disparities Roadmap, 2nd ed.* Springer Science + Business Media, New York, NY.

San Antonio, TX, USA   Amelie G. Ramirez
San Antonio, TX, USA   Ian M. Thompson
Harlingen, TX, USA   Leonel Vela

Editors

The University of Texas Health Science Center at San Antonio
Institute for Health Promotion Research (IHPR)

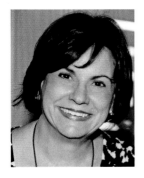

Amelie G. Ramirez, DrPH
Director, Institute for Health Promotion Research
Dielmann Chair in Health Disparities Research &
Community Outreach
Max and Minnie Tomerlin Voelcker Endowed Chair in
Cancer Health Care Disparities
Professor of Epidemiology & Biostatistics
School of Medicine
UT Health Science Center at San Antonio
7411 John Smith Drive Suite 1000
San Antonio, TX 78229, USA
http://ihpr.uthscsa.edu/

Cancer Therapy and Research Center (CTRC)

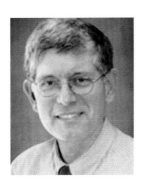

Ian M. Thompson, MD
Director, CTRC
Professor, Department of Urology
UT Health Science Center at San Antonio
Cancer Therapy and Research Center
7979 Wurzbach Rd
San Antonio, TX 78229, USA
http://thompsoni@uthscsa.edu

Regional Academic Health Center (RAHC)

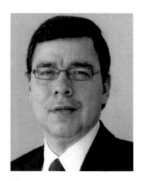

Leonel Vela, MD
Regional Dean, RAHC
Regional Academic Health Center
UT Health Science Center at San Antonio
2102 Treasure Hills Blvd.
Harlingen, TX 78550, USA

Executive Summary

South Texas, defined as the 38-county area encompassing the Texas–Mexico border counties from Cameron County to Val Verde County, as well as Bexar County (includes San Antonio), Webb County (includes Laredo), and the Lower Rio Grande Valley (Cameron, Willacy, Hidalgo, and Starr counties), is home to a unique population. In 2010, almost 4.5 million people resided in South Texas, almost 18 % of the entire Texas population, more than two-thirds of whom were Hispanic. Compared to the rest of Texas, this population is less educated, has a lower per capita personal income, and has less access to health care. Almost 30 % of South Texas adults are uninsured.

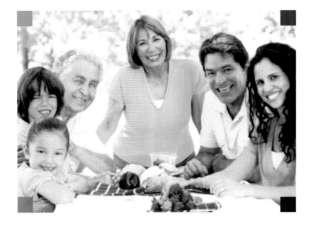

This *South Texas Health Status Review* focuses on the health of South Texas residents and explores whether there are health disparities—differences in incidence, prevalence, mortality, and burden of diseases and other adverse health conditions—among different populations within South Texas or between people who live in South Texas and people who live in the rest of Texas or nation.

This *Review* examines more than 35 health status indicators related to disease incidence and mortality, as well as behavioral factors that might put individuals at an increased risk of disease or premature mortality. These health status indicators and behavioral factors were selected because of potential disparities and, more importantly, because prevention strategies exist for most of these indicators.

For 12 of the health conditions studied, South Texas was at a disadvantage compared to the rest of Texas. For 16 health conditions, incidence/mortality rates or prevalence of conditions in South Texas were either lower than or the same as in the rest of Texas. For many health conditions, there was a greater occurrence of disease in Hispanics compared to non-Hispanic whites in South Texas. For 11 health conditions, Hispanics in South Texas had higher rates than Hispanics in the rest of Texas.

The serious conditions for which South Texas had a higher incidence or prevalence than the rest of Texas were:

- Tuberculosis
- Chlamydia
- Cervical cancer
- Liver cancer
- Stomach cancer
- Gallbladder cancer
- Child and adolescent leukemia
- Neural tube defects
- Other birth defects (common truncus and pyloric stenosis)
- Adult diabetes
- Adult obesity
- Childhood lead poisoning

The health conditions for which South Texas had lower incidence/mortality rates or prevalence than in the rest of Texas were:

- HIV/AIDS
- Syphilis
- Gonorrhea
- Breast cancer
- Colorectal cancer
- Prostate cancer
- Lung cancer
- Infant mortality
- Heart disease mortality
- Cerebrovascular disease mortality (stroke)
- Adult current asthma
- Occupational pesticide exposure
- Motor vehicle crash mortality
- Suicide mortality

Several modifiable risk factors—such as nutrition, reproductive factors, and access to health care—contribute to the differences in mortality, incidence, or prevalence experienced in South Texas, particularly among Hispanics. For example, South Texas women were less likely to have had an up-to-date Pap test than women in the rest of Texas; this lack of screening likely contributes to the higher incidence of primary cervical cancer in South Texas. Many of the observed health disparities likely are worsened by the higher percentage of people in South Texas with no health insurance.

The high prevalence of adult obesity and adult diabetes in South Texas was particularly noteworthy. South Texas had a higher prevalence of both adult obesity and diabetes than either the rest of Texas or the nation. Even among Hispanics, who have a higher prevalence of these two health conditions than non-Hispanic whites, those living in South Texas were at higher risk than Hispanics living elsewhere. Obesity, a causal risk factor for diabetes, can be directly linked to lifestyle behaviors such as inadequate physical activity and poor eating habits. Among all of the health conditions examined, obesity had the greatest impact on people (in terms of persons affected per 100,000 population) living in South Texas. Diabetes had the second greatest estimated burden on the people of South Texas. Prevention research efforts directed at obesity and diabetes could significantly reduce the burden of disease in South Texas communities.

 The high prevalence of adult obesity and adult diabetes in South Texas was particularly noteworthy. South Texas had a higher prevalence of both adult obesity and diabetes than either the rest of Texas or the nation.

Acknowledgments

The UT Health Science Center at San Antonio would like to extend its extreme gratitude to the team at the Texas Department of State Health Services (DSHS) for collating and analyzing the current South Texas, Texas, and national data on a variety of health indicators: Katie Tengelsen, MPH; Heather M. Powell; and Mark A. Canfield, PhD.

We would also like to thank the following individuals: Marc Montrose, Ann Barnett, MS, and Christopher Webb, MPH at the Center for Health Statistics; Michelle L. Cook, PhD, MPH at the Texas Behavioral Risk Factor Surveillance System; Sarah Novello, MHS at the TB/HIV/STD Epidemiology and Surveillance Branch; Rochelle Kingsley, MPH at the Pregnancy Risk Assessment Monitoring System; Cheryl L Bowcock, MPH, Lisa Marengo, MS, Reynaldo J. Velázquez, BA, L.J. Smith, MS, Jose Velez, MCSE, and Susan L. Prosperie, MS, RS—representing various programs in the Environmental Epidemiology and Disease Registries Section at the Texas DSHS; and Francisco Gonzales-Scarano, MD, Dean of the School of Medicine at the UT Health Science Center at San Antonio.

Preparation of this book was supported by the CTRC (2 P30 CA054174-17), the RAHC, and the IHPR.

Contents

Contributors

Natalie Archer Environmental Epidemiology and Disease Registries Section, Texas Department of State Health Services, Austin, TX, USA

Kipling J. Gallion Institute for Health Promotion Research, UT Health Science Center at San Antonio, San Antonio, TX, USA

Alan E.C. Holden Institute for Health Promotion Research, UT Health Science Center at San Antonio, San Antonio, TX, USA

Edgar Muñoz Institute for Health Promotion Research, UT Health Science Center at San Antonio, San Antonio, TX, USA

Dorothy Long Parma Institute for Health Promotion Research, UT Health Science Center at San Antonio, San Antonio, TX, USA

Lucina Suarez Environmental Epidemiology and Disease Registries Section, Texas Department of State Health Services, Austin, TX, USA

Chapter 1
Introduction

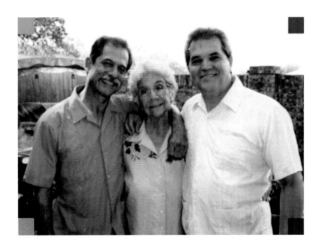

The majority of individuals in South Texas are of Hispanic ethnicity (68.9 % in 2010) [1]. Hispanics typically face a number of barriers to health care including economic, cultural, and institutional barriers. Inadequate access to health care may lead to disparities in health outcomes [2, 3].

This report focuses on the health of South Texas residents by analyzing nearly 40 health status indicators to determine if disparities exist either between South Texans and those residing in the nation, the rest of Texas or among different populations within South Texas. The indicators in this document measure health status, mortality, and behavioral factors that might heighten individuals' risk of disease or premature mortality.

A.G. Ramirez et al. (eds.), *The South Texas Health Status Review:*
A Health Disparities Roadmap, DOI 10.1007/978-3-319-00233-0_1, © The Author(s) 2013

Overview

In this chapter, South Texas is defined as a 38-county, 45,926-square-mile area (Fig. 1.1) [4]. The area contains many counties along the Texas–Mexico border, from Cameron County (in southernmost Texas) northwest to Val Verde County.

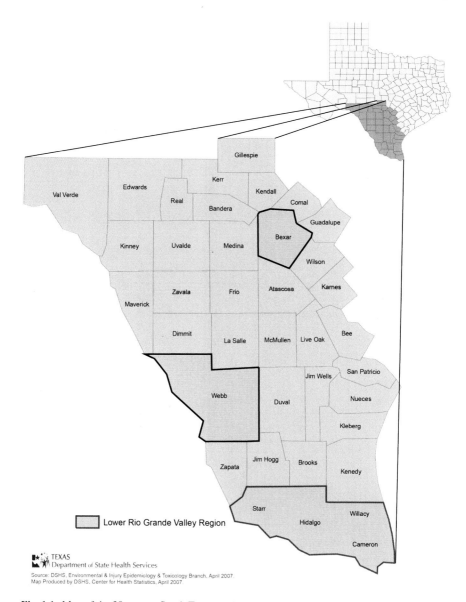

Fig. 1.1 Map of the 38-county South Texas study area

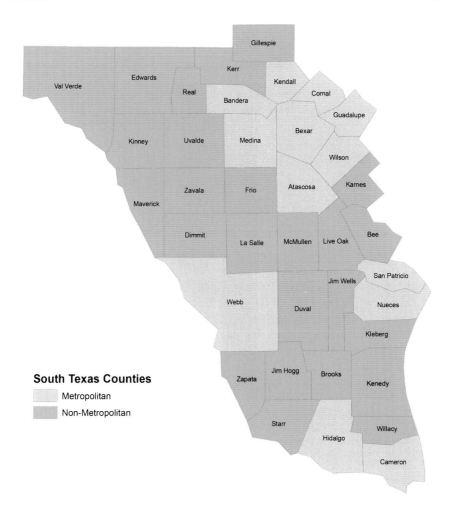

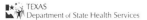

Source: DSHS, Environmental & Injury Epidemiology & Toxicology Branch, April 2007.
Map Produced by DSHS, Center for Health Statistics, April 2007.

Fig. 1.2 Map of metropolitan and nonmetropolitan counties in South Texas, as designated by the U.S. Office of Management and Budget, 2003, OMB Bulletin No. 03–04

The area also contains Bexar County (including San Antonio), Webb County (including Laredo), and the Lower Rio Grande Valley (a group of four counties— Cameron, Willacy, Hidalgo, and Starr—that were sometimes analyzed separately from the rest of South Texas).

Of the 38 counties covered in this chapter, 13 are considered metropolitan and 25 are considered nonmetropolitan (Fig. 1.2). A metropolitan county has a core urban area with a population of 50,000 or more. Any adjacent counties with a high degree of economic and social integration with the core urban area are also designated metropolitan [5]. Counties not meeting these criteria are designated nonmetropolitan.

In 2011, almost 4.5 million people resided in South Texas. Estimated county populations ranged from 470 residents in Kenedy County to more than 1.6 million in Bexar County [1]. The average population density for South Texas was 268.8 persons per square mile in metropolitan counties and 17 persons per square mile in nonmetropolitan counties [1, 4].

Study Goals

The goal of this study is to examine a number of health status indicators to determine if disparities exist between the South Texas population and the population in the rest of Texas, between South Texas and the nation, and/or among South Texas subpopulations. This study identifies possible health disparities and makes recommendations about where to focus public health efforts.

The health status indicators analyzed in this chapter are listed in Table 1.1. These health status indicators were chosen because of potential disparities between the South Texas area and the rest of Texas and nation, and, more importantly, because prevention strategies exist for most of these indicators.

Table 1.1 List of health status indicators analyzed in this document

Health status indicators		
Communicable diseases	*Cancer incidence/mortality*	*Maternal and child health*
Tuberculosis	Breast cancer	Prenatal care
HIV/AIDS	Cervical cancer	Preconception health care
Syphilis	Colorectal cancer	Unintended pregnancy
Gonorrhea	Prostate cancer	Preconception overweight
Chlamydia	Lung cancer	and obesity
	Liver cancer	Birth defects
		Infant mortality
Chronic diseases	Stomach cancer	
Diabetes	Gallbladder cancer	*Behavioral risk factors*
Heart disease mortality	Child/adolescent leukemia	Obesity
Stroke mortality		Nutrition
Asthma	*Injury*	Physical activity
	Motor vehicle crash mortality	Smoking behaviors
Environmental factors	Homicide	Alcohol use
Childhood lead poisoning	Suicide	Cancer screening
Pesticide exposures		

References

1. Texas Department of State Health Services. Texas health data: population. http://soupfin.tdh. state.tx.us/pop2000a.htm. Accessed June 2012.
2. US Department of Health and Human Services, Agency for Healthcare Research and Quality. National healthcare disparities report. 2011. AHRQ Publication No. 12–0006. 2012.
3. Scheppers E, van Dongen E, Dekker J, Geertzen J, Dekker J. Potential barriers to the use of health services among ethnic minorities: a review. Fam Pract. 2006;23:325–48.
4. United States Census Bureau. State and county quickfacts – Texas. http://quickfacts.census. gov/qfd/states/48000.html. Accessed June 2012.
5. Office of Information and Regulatory Affairs, Office of Management and Budget, Executive Office of the President. Office of Management and Budget: 2010 standards for defining metropolitan and micropolitan statistical areas. Fed Regist. 2010;75:37246–52.

Chapter 2
South Texas Population Characteristics

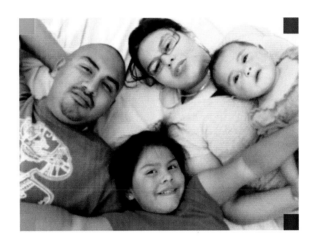

Almost 4.5 million people were estimated to have resided in South Texas in 2010, almost 18 % of the entire Texas population. From 2000 to 2010, South Texas grew at the same rate as the rest of Texas. However, the population growth rates among specific races/ethnicities differed slightly between South Texas and the rest of Texas (Table 2.1). Metropolitan counties in South Texas experienced more population growth between 2000 and 2010 (an average of 23.6 %) than did nonmetropolitan counties (10.7 %). The five fastest-growing South Texas counties from 2000 to 2010 were Comal, Kendall, Guadalupe, Wilson, and Hidalgo counties [1].

In 2010, 68.9 % of the South Texas population was estimated to be Hispanic, 25.2 % was non-Hispanic white, and 3.9 % was African-American. In the rest of Texas, Hispanics comprised only 32.4 % of the population, with non-Hispanic whites clearly the majority, making up 49.3 % of the population. Also, a much larger percentage of the rest of Texas population (13.2 %) was African-American (Table 2.2) [1].

A.G. Ramirez et al. (eds.), *The South Texas Health Status Review:*
A Health Disparities Roadmap, DOI 10.1007/978-3-319-00233-0_2, © The Author(s) 2013

Table 2.1 Percent estimated population growth between 2000 and 2010 in South Texas and the rest of Texas, by race/ethnicity

Location	Race/ethnicity	2000 Population	2010 Population	% Population growth
South Texas	All Races	3,669,885	4,473,918	21.9
	White	1,114,742	1,127,594	1.2
	Black	135,438	172,789	27.6
	Hispanic	2,369,796	3,080,387	30.0
	Other	49,909	93,148	86.6
Rest of Texas	All Races	17,181,935	20,900,029	21.6
	White	9,959,974	10,314,001	3.6
	Black	2,286,215	2,752,962	20.4
	Hispanic	4,299,870	6,767,465	57.4
	Other	635,876	1,065,601	67.6

Source: Texas Health Data (http://soupfin.tdh.state.tx.us/people.htm); 2000 Census data and 2010 projection data were used

Table 2.2 Race/ethnic breakdown of the projected South Texas and rest of Texas populations, 2010

Race	South Texas (%)	Rest of Texas (%)
Non-Hispanic White	25.2	49.3
Hispanic	68.9	32.4
African-American	3.9	13.2
Other	2.1	5.1

Source: Texas Health Data (http://soupfin.tdh.state.tx.us/people. htm); 2010 projection data were used

The age distribution of the South Texas population in 2010 is shown in Fig. 2.1. The South Texas population as a whole is slightly younger than the rest of Texas. Almost 40 % of individuals in South Texas are younger than age 25 (Fig. 2.1).

Overall, the adult South Texas population is slightly less educated than the total Texas population. In South Texas in 2006–2010, 73.9 % of the population age 25 or older were high school graduates (compared to 80 % of Texas overall) and 20.5 % had a bachelors' degree or higher (compared to 25.8 % in Texas overall) [2]. South Texas residents' per capita personal income in 2010 was lower than for all of Texas, and the poverty rate in South Texas was higher (Table 2.3) [3, 4]. In 2010, 8.9 % of the South Texas population was unemployed, and 23.6 % lived below the poverty level. During this same time period, Texas' unemployment rate was 8.2 % and poverty rate was 17.9 % [4, 5]. The top 10 counties with the highest poverty rates in Texas in 2010 were all South Texas counties, ranging from 32.3 % (Zapata) to 39.9 % (Maverick) [4].

Approximately 98 % of South Texans are on public water systems, and 75 % of the population served by these systems receives fluoridated water [6].

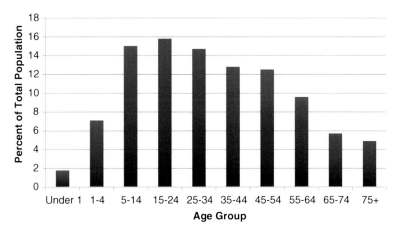

Fig. 2.1 Population age trends in South Texas, 2010. *Source*: Texas Health Data (http://soupfin. tdh.state.tx.us/people.htm); 2010 projection data were used

Table 2.3 Socioeconomic statistics for South Texas and all of Texas

Socioeconomic Indicator	South Texas	All of Texas
Education:		
% High school grad or higher, 2006–2010	73.9	80.0
% Bachelor's degree or higher, 2000	20.5	25.8
Per capita personal income, 2010	$30,135	$37,747
Unemployment rate, 2010	8.9 %	8.2 %
Poverty rate, 2010	23.6 %	17.9 %

Source: Education indicators: American Community Survey 5-year estimates; per capita personal income: US Department of Commerce; unemployment: US Bureau of Labor Statistics; poverty rates: US Census Bureau

References

1. Texas Department of State Health Services. Texas health data: population. http://soupfin.tdh. state.tx.us/pop2000a.htm. Accessed June 2012.
2. US Census Bureau. American community survey 2006–2010 5-year estimates, Table B15. 2011. http://factfinder.census.gov/. Accessed Apr 2012.
3. Bureau of Economic Analysis, U.S. Department of Commerce. Regional data – GDP and personal income. 2012. http://www.bea.gov/iTable/iTable.cfm?ReqID=70&step=1. Accessed July 2012.
4. US Census Bureau. Small area income and poverty estimates. 2012. http://www.census.gov// did/www/saipe/index.html. Accessed May 2012.
5. Bureau of Labor Statistics, U.S. Department of Labor. Local area unemployment statistics. 2012. Accessed July 2012.
6. Centers for Disease Control and Prevention. 2010. Water Fluoridation Statistics. http://www. cdc.gov/fluoridation/statistics/2010stats.htm. Last updated July 27, 2012. Accessed May 2013.

Chapter 3
Access to Health Care in South Texas

Adequate access to health care services, including preventive services and treatment for illnesses, is critical to achieving positive health outcomes. Two major limitations of adequate access to care are a lack of health insurance coverage and a shortage of health care providers in certain areas [1, 2].

Lack of Health Insurance

Lack of health insurance coverage is a significant barrier to seeking and receiving health care [2, 3]. Nationwide, Hispanics and young adults aged 18–24 are more likely to be uninsured than other demographic groups [1, 4].

Using Texas Behavioral Risk Factor Surveillance System (BRFSS) survey data, an estimated 30 % of South Texas adult residents were uninsured during 2007–2010. South Texas had a higher percentage of uninsured residents than the rest of Texas (23 %). Both South Texas and the rest of Texas had a higher percentage of uninsured residents than the nationwide BRFSS estimate of about 15 % (Fig. 3.1). During 2007–2010, the estimated South Texas uninsured rate was almost twice as high as the national rate.

In South Texas during 2007–2010, Hispanics and African-Americans had higher percentages of uninsured individuals than did non-Hispanic whites. South Texas Hispanics had the highest uninsured rate (40.8 %) of all race/ethnic groups. The percentage of Hispanics with no health care was almost 3.5 times higher than for non-Hispanic whites, and twice as high for African Americans (Fig. 3.2).

In 2007–2010, estimates indicate that half of adults aged 18–29 in South Texas had no health insurance (Fig. 3.3), the highest rate among all age groups. The percentage of individuals with no health insurance dropped steadily with age (Fig. 3.3).

A.G. Ramirez et al. (eds.), *The South Texas Health Status Review:*
A Health Disparities Roadmap, DOI 10.1007/978-3-319-00233-0_3, © The Author(s) 2013

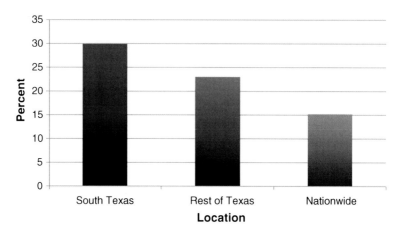

Fig. 3.1 Estimated percent of the adult population (18+) with no health insurance by location, 2007–2010. *Source*: Texas Behavioral Risk Factor Surveillance System Combined Year Dataset, Statewide BRFSS Survey, 2007–2010

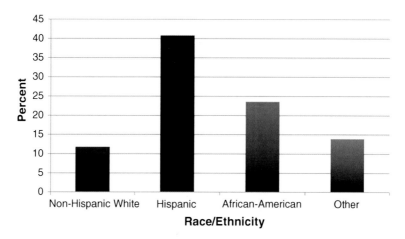

Fig. 3.2 Estimated percent of adult (18+) South Texas population with no health insurance by race/ethnicity, 2007–2010. *Source*: Texas Behavioral Risk Factor Surveillance System Combined Year Dataset, Statewide BRFSS Survey, 2007–2010

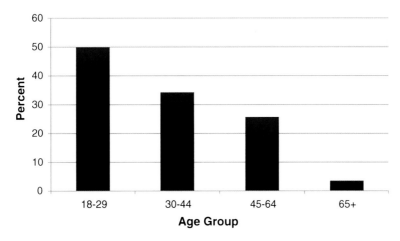

Fig. 3.3 Estimated percent of the adult (18+) South Texas population with no health insurance by age group, 2007–2010. *Source*: Texas Behavioral Risk Factor Surveillance System Combined Year Dataset, Statewide BRFSS Survey, 2007–2010

Health Professional Shortage Areas

Another major barrier to receiving adequate health care is a shortage of health care providers in certain locations. Twenty-four of the 38 South Texas counties are currently designated by the U.S. Department of Health and Human Services as (whole county service area) primary care health professional shortage areas (HPSAs) [5].

The counties designated as primary care HPSAs in South Texas are shown in Fig. 3.4. The HPSAs in this list are mostly nonmetropolitan counties. However, a few metropolitan counties (such as Atascosa, Bandera, Medina, and Wilson) are designated as HPSAs, so a shortage of health professionals is also a problem in some South Texas metropolitan areas [5].

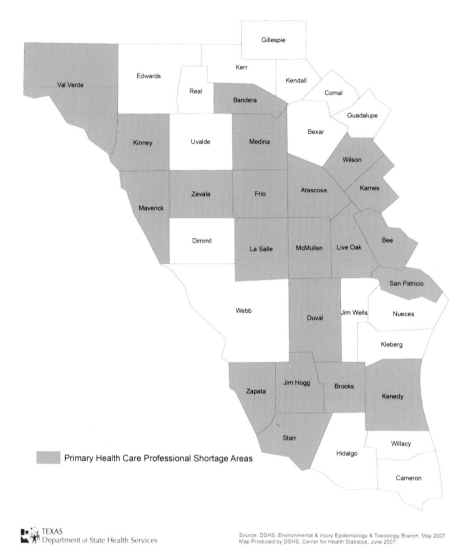

Fig. 3.4 Map of designated whole county primary care health professional shortage areas in South Texas, 2010

References

1. Zuvekas SH, Weinick RM. Changes in access to care, 1977–1996: the role of health insurance. Health Serv Res. 1999;34:271–9.
2. Healthy People 2020. Access to health services. 2012. http://1.usa.gov/f8uTOp. Accessed June 2012.
3. Weinick RM, Zuvekas SH, Drilea S. Research findings #3: access to health care – sources and barriers, 1996. Agency for Healthcare Research and Quality. 2006. http://www.meps.ahrq.gov/mepsweb/data_files/publications/rf3/rf3.shtml. Accessed 2007 Apr 2007.
4. U.S. Department of Health and Human Services. Overview of the uninsured in the United States: a summary of the 2011 current population survey. 2011. http://aspe.hhs.gov/health/reports/2011/CPSHealthIns2011/ib.shtml. Accessed June 2012.
5. UU.S. Department of Health and Human Services, Health Resources and Services Administration. Find shortage areas: APSA by state and county. 2012. http://hpsafind.hrsa.gov/HPSASearch.aspx. Accessed May 2012.. Accessed June 2012.

Chapter 4
Communicable Diseases

A communicable disease is one that can be transmitted or spread from one person or species to another, through either direct or indirect contact [1]. A multitude of different communicable diseases are currently reportable in Texas including tuberculosis and many types of sexually transmitted diseases. Incidence rates for communicable diseases in this chapter are presented as crude rates, without age-adjustment.

Tuberculosis

Tuberculosis (TB) is a chronic infection caused by the *Mycobacterium tuberculosis* bacterium. Although most people infected with *M. tuberculosis* harbor the bacterium with no symptoms (latent TB), some people do eventually develop active TB disease. TB is spread from person to person through the air. Only people with active TB disease can spread the bacteria to others [2]. TB usually affects the lungs, although it sometimes can also affect other parts of the body such as the brain, the kidneys, or the spine. TB disease can cause serious health problems, including death, if left untreated [2].

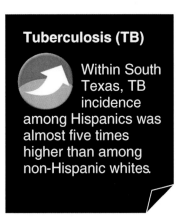

Tuberculosis (TB)

Within South Texas, TB incidence among Hispanics was almost five times higher than among non-Hispanic whites.

A total of 11,181 TB cases were reported in the USA in 2010 [3]. In addition to these active TB cases, more than 11 million people in the USA are estimated to currently have latent TB infection [4]. TB incidence in the USA was much higher among African-Americans (7.0/100,000), Asians (22.5/100,000), and Hispanics (6.5/100,000) than among non-Hispanic whites (0.9/100,000) in 2010 [3]. Nationwide, males have a higher risk of TB

A.G. Ramirez et al. (eds.), *The South Texas Health Status Review:*
A Health Disparities Roadmap, DOI 10.1007/978-3-319-00233-0_4, © The Author(s) 2013

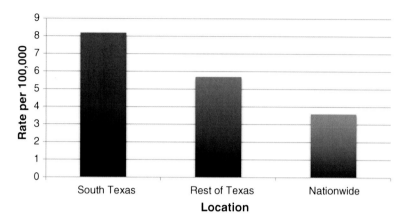

Fig. 4.1 Incidence of active tuberculosis (TB) disease by location. *Source*: Texas data: TB/HIV/ STD Epidemiology and Surveillance Branch, Texas Department of State Health Services, 2006– 2010. Nationwide data is for 2010 only, obtained from Pratt et al. 2011 [3]

disease than females, and people in older age groups are more at risk for TB than people of younger ages [5]. Foreign-born persons are also disproportionately affected by TB. In 2010, the incidence of TB disease was 11 times higher among foreign-born persons in the USA than among persons born in the USA [3]. A TB infection can develop into active TB disease as a result of conditions or exposures that can reduce a person's immunity such as HIV infection, diabetes, or chemo-therapy treatment. Other risk factors for TB include low income, long-term drug or alcohol use, and living or working in prisons or nursing homes [6].

Tuberculosis in South Texas

The incidence of active TB disease in South Texas during 2006–2010 was 8.2/100,000, a higher incidence of TB than individuals living in the rest of Texas and nationwide (Fig. 4.1). The 2006–2010 average annual incidence of TB in South Texas was 2.3 times higher than the TB rate reported nationwide in 2010.

Hispanics in South Texas had a higher incidence of TB (10.2/100,000) than did Hispanics in the rest of Texas (7.3/100,000) in 2006–2010. TB incidence among South Texas Hispanics was almost five times higher than the incidence among non-Hispanic whites (Fig. 4.2).

Among Hispanics, the TB incidence increased sharply with age, in contrast with a more gradual age increase among non-Hispanic whites (Fig. 4.3). Hispanics aged 45 or older had the highest TB incidence, 17.4/100,000.

Males in South Texas had an incidence of TB more than twice as high as the incidence in females. When stratifying by sex and race/ethnicity, TB incidence

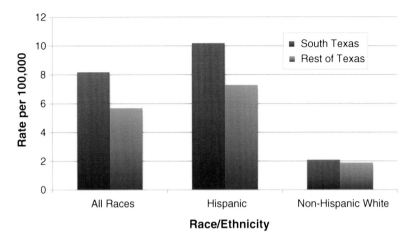

Fig. 4.2 Incidence of active tuberculosis (TB) by location and race/ethnicity, 2006–2010. *Source:* TB/HIV/STD Epidemiology and Surveillance Branch, Texas Department of State Health Services

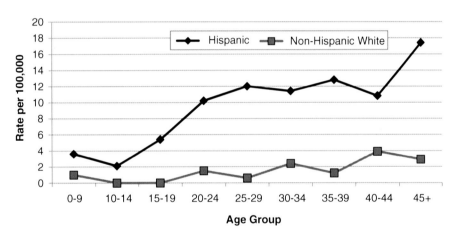

Fig. 4.3 Incidence of tuberculosis in South Texas by age group and race/ethnicity, 2006–2010. *Source:* TB/HIV/STD Epidemiology and Surveillance Branch, Texas Department of State Health Services

estimates ranged from 14.0/100,000 in Hispanic males to 1.1/100,000 in non-Hispanic white females (Fig. 4.4).

In 2006–2010, the incidence of TB in Bexar County (5.3/100,000) was lower than the incidence in South Texas as a whole (8.2/100,000). However, TB estimates in Webb County (15.2/100,000) and the four-county Lower Rio Grande Valley region (12.3/100,000) were 1.5–2 times higher than in all of South Texas (Fig. 4.5).

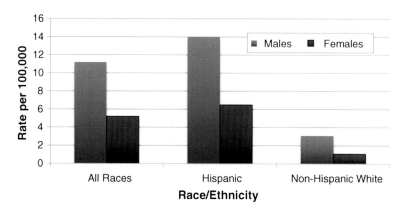

Fig. 4.4 Incidence of tuberculosis in South Texas by sex and race/ethnicity, 2006–2010. *Source*: TB/HIV/STD Epidemiology and Surveillance Branch, Texas Department of State Health Services

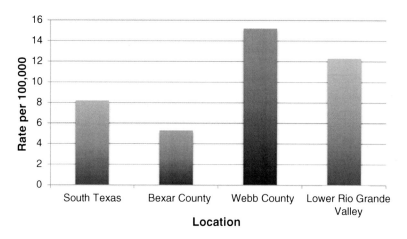

Fig. 4.5 Incidence of tuberculosis in selected South Texas locations, 2006–2010. *Source*: TB/HIV/STD Epidemiology and Surveillance Branch, Texas Department of State Health Services

HIV/AIDS

HIV (human immunodeficiency virus) is a human retrovirus that infects and slowly depletes a type of white blood cells known as T-lymphocytes or CD^{4+} T-lymphocytes. These white blood cells are essential to maintaining an effective immune response. HIV gradually destroys the body's ability to fight infections and certain cancers by damaging or killing immune system cells [7]. People with HIV have what is called HIV infection. Some of these people will develop AIDS (acquired immunodeficiency syndrome) as a result of their HIV infection [7]. HIV is most commonly transmitted by having unprotected sex with a partner who is infected. HIV can also be spread through contact with infected blood such as sharing drug needles or syringes or through contaminated blood transfusions. Women infected with HIV can transmit the virus to their babies during pregnancy or birth or through breast milk [8].

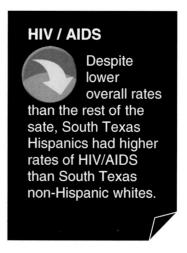

HIV / AIDS

Despite lower overall rates than the rest of the sate, South Texas Hispanics had higher rates of HIV/AIDS than South Texas non-Hispanic whites.

Many people do not have any symptoms when they first become infected with HIV. This "asymptomatic" infection period can differ greatly among individuals. Some people may begin to experience symptoms within just a few months, while others may remain symptom free for more than 10 years [8, 9]. AIDS refers to the most advanced stages of HIV infection [8]. People with AIDS often contract opportunistic infections that do not usually affect healthy people. In AIDS patients, these infections are frequently severe and are sometimes fatal, because the immune system has been so damaged by HIV that it can no longer resist bacteria, viruses, parasites, or other microbes [9]. People with AIDS are also particularly susceptible to certain cancers [10]. No cure exists for HIV or AIDS. However, a number of drugs currently exist that can slow the progression of HIV infection as well as fight associated cancers and infections [9, 10].

In 2008, approximately 1.2 million individuals in the USA were estimated to be living with either HIV or AIDS, of which an estimated 20 % were undiagnosed and unaware that they had HIV [11]. There were an estimated 17,774 AIDS deaths in the USA in 2009. The HIV/AIDS epidemic in the USA continues to disproportionately affect minority groups. The rate of new HIV infection in 2010 was more than eight times higher in African-Americans and almost three times higher in Hispanics than in non-Hispanic whites [12]. In 2009, 77 % of newly diagnosed HIV cases in the USA were male [11]. Major risk factors for HIV/AIDS include having unprotected sex with multiple partners or with men who have sex with men, sharing needles during drug use, or already having hepatitis, tuberculosis (TB), or another sexually transmitted disease (STD) such as syphilis, herpes, or chlamydia [7, 10].

HIV/AIDS in South Texas

In 2006–2010, the average annual incidence of HIV/AIDS in South Texas was 11.3/100,000, a lower rate than the incidence in the rest of Texas (18.1/100,000). Overall, the incidence of HIV/AIDS was about 60 % higher in the rest of Texas than in South Texas (Fig. 4.6). In South Texas, Hispanics had a higher incidence of HIV/AIDS (11.4/100,000) than non-Hispanic whites (8.2/100,000) (Fig. 4.6).

Fig. 4.6 Incidence of HIV/
AIDS by location and race/
ethnicity, 2006–2010. *Source*:
TB/HIV/STD Epidemiology
and Surveillance Branch,
Texas Department of State
Health Services

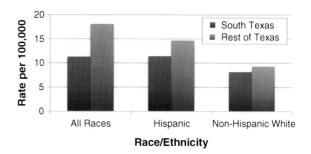

Fig. 4.7 Incidence of HIV/
AIDS in selected South Texas
locations, 2006–2010.
Source: TB/HIV/STD
Epidemiology and
Surveillance Branch, Texas
Department of State Health
Services

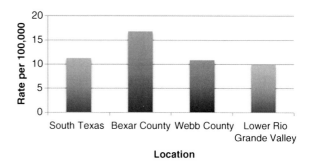

In South Texas, the incidence of HIV/AIDS was more than 4.5 times higher in males (18.8/100,000) than females (4.1/100,000). Individuals aged 20–44 had significantly higher rates of HIV/AIDS than other age groups. The incidence of HIV/AIDS was about two times higher in South Texas metropolitan counties (12.1/100,000) than in nonmetropolitan counties (5.8/100,000). Bexar County had a higher incidence of HIV/AIDS (16.8/100,000) than South Texas as a whole (11.3/100,000), whereas the incidence of HIV/AIDS in Webb County (9.9/100,000) was lower than that seen in all of South Texas. The incidence of HIV/AIDS in the Lower Rio Grande Valley region (10.9/100,000) was similar to the incidence in South Texas as a whole (Fig. 4.7).

Syphilis

Syphilis is a sexually transmitted disease (STD) caused by the *Treponema pallidum* bacterium. Syphilis has been called "the great imitator" because many possible symptoms are associated with the disease, and these symptoms often mirror ones seen in many other diseases [13, 14]. Syphilis is most commonly spread by sexual contact with an infected individual [13]. The syphilis bacterium is transmitted by direct contact with a syphilis sore; sores usually occur on the genitals or anus but can also occur on the lips or in the mouth. Syphilis *can also be transmitted from an infected mother to her baby during pregnancy* [14]. The primary stage of syphilis is character- ized by one or more small, round sores, called chancres, that are located where the bacterium entered the body. Because chancres are usually not painful, can occur inside the body, and heal without treatment, symptoms of primary syphi- lis may go unnoticed. If left untreated, the syphi- lis infection progresses to the secondary stage, which is usually marked by a skin rash. Symptoms of secondary syphilis may be mild and will also go away without treatment. However, without treatment, syphilis infection is still present in the body. Although there may be no outward signs or symptoms for many years after secondary syphilis, untreated syphi- lis infection may damage internal organs such as the heart, brain, nervous system, eyes, bones,

Syphilis

Despite lower overall rates than the rest of the state, the incidence of syphilis among South Texas Hispanics was more than two times higher than South Texas non-Hispanic whites.

and joints. Late-stage syphilis infection, which occurs in about 15 % of untreated individuals, can cause blindness, deafness, mental illness, paralysis, heart disease, and even death [13, 14]. Untreated syphilis in pregnant women is associated with a high risk of adverse pregnancy outcomes such as miscarriage, stillbirth, preterm birth, and infant mortality [14, 15]. Syphilis is curable with antibiotics, but treat- ment cannot repair damage already done to the body by syphilis infection [14].

In 2010, 45,834 new cases of syphilis (at all stages) were reported in the USA including 13,774 cases of primary and secondary syphilis. Nationwide, the inci- dence of primary and secondary syphilis was seven times higher among men than among women in 2010. The incidence of primary and secondary syphilis in the USA was eight times higher among African-Americans and two times higher among Hispanics than among non-Hispanic whites [16]. The age-specific incidence of syphilis in the USA varied depending on race/ethnicity and sex, although among both Hispanic and non-Hispanic white women, the highest incidence of primary and secondary syphilis was observed among those aged 20–24 [15]. Men who have unprotected sex with other men have a higher risk of syphilis infection than the general population [16, 17]. Other risk factors for syphilis include having unpro- tected sex and having sex with multiple partners [13, 17].

Syphilis in South Texas

Overall, the average annual incidence of syphilis (all stages) during 2006–2010 was lower in South Texas (19.8/100,000) than in the rest of Texas (25.9/100,000). However, Hispanics in South Texas had a higher incidence of syphilis (21.9/100,000)

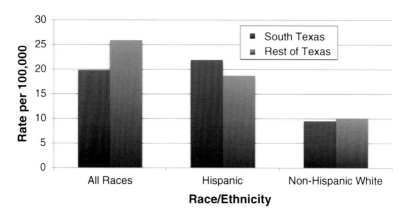

Fig. 4.8 Incidence of syphilis by location and race/ethnicity, 2006–2010. *Source*: TB/HIV/STD Epidemiology and Surveillance Branch, Texas Department of State Health Services

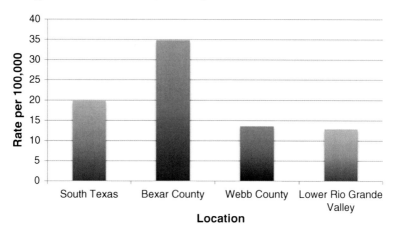

Fig. 4.9 Incidence of syphilis in selected South Texas locations, 2006–2010. *Source*: TB/HIV/ STD Epidemiology and Surveillance Branch, Texas Department of State Health Services

than did Hispanics in the rest of Texas (18.7/100,000). In South Texas, the incidence of syphilis among Hispanics was more than two times higher than the incidence among non-Hispanic whites (Fig. 4.8).

South Texas females had a much lower incidence of syphilis (13.3/100,000) than males (26.4/100,000). The incidence of syphilis in South Texas was highest among individuals aged 20–29 (more than 45/100,000). Syphilis incidence was about three times higher in South Texas metropolitan counties (21.5/100,000) than in nonmetropolitan counties (7.2/100,000) in 2006–2010. The incidence of syphilis was higher in Bexar County (34.8/100,000) than in South Texas as a whole (19.8/100,000) in 2006–2010. However, syphilis incidence was lower in Webb County (13.6/100,000) and in the Lower Rio Grande Valley region (12.9/100,000) compared to all of South Texas during this timeframe (Fig. 4.9).

Chlamydia

Chlamydia is a sexually transmitted disease (STD) caused by the *Chlamydia trachomatis* bacterium. Chlamydia bacteria live in vaginal fluid and semen *and can be transmitted to a partner during vaginal, anal, or oral sex. Chlamydia can also be transmitted from an infected mother to her infant during a vaginal childbirth.* Chlamydia can also be found in the throat, and eyes in both sexes [18, 19]. Individuals frequently do not know that they are infected with chlamydia, because symptoms of chlamydia are often mild or completely absent. *This is problematic, because if left untreated, chlamydia infection can cause irreversible reproductive and other health problems, particularly in women* [18]. *Chlamydia is the most frequently reported notifiable disease in America,* with more than 1.3 million cases reported in 2010 [16, 18]. However, because most individuals are unaware that they have chlamydia and thus do not get tested, underreporting of this disease is considerable. It is estimated that 2.8 million persons in the USA are actually infected with chlamydia every year [18].

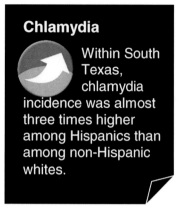

Chlamydia

Within South Texas, chlamydia incidence was almost three times higher among Hispanics than among non-Hispanic whites.

In 2010, the reported incidence of chlamydia infection among women in the USA was more than two-and-a-half times higher than the incidence among men, most likely because a greater number of women are screened for chlamydia than men. Among US women, the highest age-specific chlamydia incidence was observed among those aged 15–24, while age-specific incidence of chlamydia in men was highest among those aged 20–24 [16]. If sexually active, teenage girls and young women are at higher risk of chlamydia infection than older women, because the cervix has not yet fully matured [18].

Nationwide, the incidence of chlamydia among African-Americans is more than eight times higher than the incidence among non-Hispanic whites. Chlamydia incidence is also more than four times higher among Native Americans and nearly three times higher among Hispanics than among non-Hispanic whites [16]. Other risk factors for chlamydia include having unprotected sex and having multiple sex partners [18].

Chlamydia in South Texas

The average annual incidence of chlamydia in South Texas was 429.4/100,000 in 2006–2010, a higher rate than the incidence of chlamydia in the rest of Texas (387.4/100,000). Although Hispanics also had a higher incidence of chlamydia in South Texas than in the rest of Texas, for non-Hispanic whites, incidence in South Texas was similar to the incidence in the rest of Texas (Fig. 4.9).

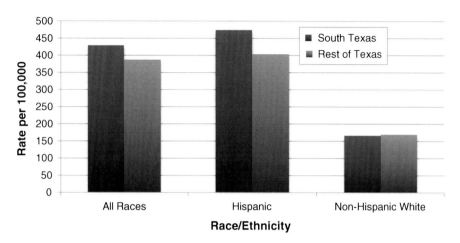

Fig. 4.10 Incidence of chlamydia by location and race/ethnicity, 2006–2010. *Source*: TB/HIV/STD Epidemiology and Surveillance Branch, Texas Department of State Health Services

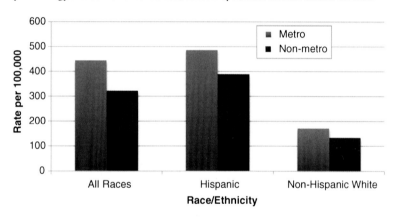

Fig. 4.11 Incidence of chlamydia in South Texas by county designation and race/ethnicity, 2006–2010. *Source*: TB/HIV/STD Epidemiology and Surveillance Branch, Texas Department of State Health Services

Chlamydia incidence was almost three times higher among Hispanics than among non-Hispanic whites in South Texas (Fig. 4.10).

The incidence of chlamydia among South Texas females (666.3/100,000) was more than 3.5 times higher than the incidence among males (185.8/100,000). As observed nationwide, individuals aged 15–24 had a much higher incidence of chlamydia than any other age groups. In South Texas, individuals aged 20–24 had an incidence of 1,970.7/100,000.

Overall, chlamydia incidence was significantly higher in South Texas metropolitan counties (443.9/100,000) than nonmetropolitan counties (322.2/100,000) (Fig. 4.11).

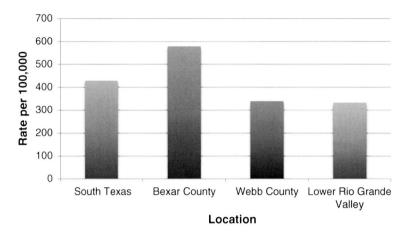

Fig. 4.12 Incidence of chlamydia in selected South Texas locations, 2006–2010. *Source*: TB/HIV/STD Epidemiology and Surveillance Branch, Texas Department of State Health Services

In 2006–2010, the incidence of chlamydia was higher in Bexar County (578.5/100,000) than in South Texas as a whole (429.4/100,000). However, chlamydia incidence estimates were lower in Webb County (340/100,000) and the Lower Rio Grande Valley region (333.5/100,000) than in South Texas (Fig. 4.12).

Gonorrhea

Gonorrhea is a sexually transmitted disease (STD) caused by the *Neisseria gonorrhoeae* bacterium. This bacterium grows easily in many parts of the reproductive tract, including the cervix, uterus, and fallopian tubes in women, and the urinary tract in both women and men [16, 20]. Gonorrhea can also grow in the throat, mouth, eyes, and anus. Gonorrhea bacteria *can be transmitted by contact with the penis, mouth, vagina, or anus of an infected individual; ejaculation is not necessary for the disease to be spread. Gonorrhea can also be transmitted from an infected mother to her baby during childbirth* [20]. If left untreated, gonorrhea can cause permanent health problems in

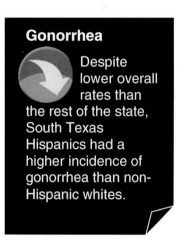

Gonorrhea

Despite lower overall rates than the rest of the state, South Texas Hispanics had a higher incidence of gonorrhea than non-Hispanic whites.

both sexes, and can cause a painful testicular condition called epididymitis in men. Untreated gonorrhea infection also appears to increase the risk of both transmitting and acquiring HIV [16, 20]. *Gonorrhea can usually be successfully treated and cured with antibiotics; however, drug-resistant gonorrhea infections are becoming more common in the U.S., making treatment more difficult* [16, 20].

Gonorrhea is the second-most frequently reported notifiable disease in the USA. There were 309,341 reported cases of gonorrhea in the USA in 2010; however, because many people with gonorrhea are asymptomatic and thus do not get tested, this disease is often underreported [16, 20]. The CDC estimates that more than 700,000 new gonorrhea infections occur each year [20]. In 2010, the Southern region of the USA, which includes Texas, had a higher incidence of gonorrhea than the other regions. Nationwide, the incidence of gonorrhea is currently slightly higher among women than men, and age-specific gonorrhea incidence is highest among women aged 15–24 and men aged 20–24 [16]. The incidence of gonorrhea is nearly 19 times higher among African-Americans, more than 4.5 times higher among Native Americans, and more than twice as high among Hispanics than among non-Hispanic whites [16]. Like most STDs, the major risk factors for gonorrhea include having unprotected sex and sex with multiple partners [20, 21].

Gonorrhea in South Texas

Overall, the average annual incidence of gonorrhea in South Texas (98.5/100,000) was much lower than the incidence of gonorrhea in the rest of Texas (132.1/100,000). Non-Hispanic whites in South Texas had a slightly lower incidence of gonorrhea than non-Hispanic whites in the rest of Texas, and Hispanics in South Texas had a higher incidence than Hispanics in the rest of Texas (Fig. 4.13). The high overall incidence of gonorrhea observed in the rest of Texas is possibly due to a higher percent of African-Americans residing in the rest of Texas than in South Texas (as African-Americans have a higher incidence of gonorrhea than any other USA racial/ethnic group).

Hispanics had a higher incidence of gonorrhea than non-Hispanic whites, both in South Texas and in the rest of Texas. In 2006–2010, the average annual incidence of gonorrhea among Hispanics in South Texas (90.3/100,000) was 2.4 times higher than among non-Hispanic whites (37.6/100,000) (Fig. 4.13).

In South Texas, the incidence of gonorrhea was higher for females (101.3/100,000) than for males (95.6/100,000). Individuals aged 20–24 had a higher risk of gonorrhea (408.2/100,000) than all other age groups in South Texas. The incidence of gonorrhea was 2.7 times higher in South Texas metropolitan counties (106.5/100,000) than nonmetropolitan counties (39.3/100,000). Bexar County had a much higher incidence of gonorrhea (185.1/100,000) than all of South Texas (98.5/100,000); however, the gonorrhea incidence estimates for Webb County (24.7/100,000) and the Lower Rio Grande Valley region (27.2/100,000) were much lower than for South Texas as a whole (Fig. 4.14). In 2006–2010, the incidence of gonorrhea in Webb County was almost four times lower than the incidence of gonorrhea in South Texas.

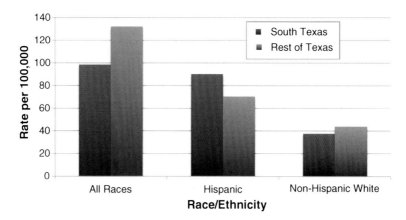

Fig. 4.13 Incidence of gonorrhea by location and race/ethnicity, 2006–2010. *Source*: TB/HIV/ STD Epidemiology and Surveillance Branch, Texas Department of State Health Services

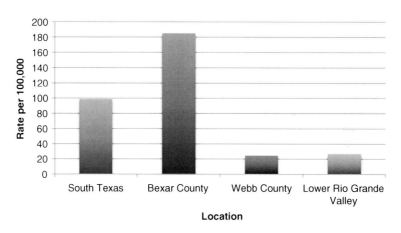

Fig. 4.14 Incidence of gonorrhea in selected South Texas locations, 2006–2010. *Source*: TB/HIV/ STD Epidemiology and Surveillance Branch, Texas Department of State Health Services

Summary

Table 4.1 Summary table of crude incidence rates in South Texas, the rest of Texas, and nationwide[a] for each of the communicable diseases analyzed

Health indicator	Incidence per 100,000 population		
	South Texas, 2001–2005	Rest of Texas, 2001–2005	Nationwide, 2010
Tuberculosis	8.2	5.7	3.6
HIV/AIDS	11.3	18.1	[b]
Syphilis	19.8	25.9	[b]
Chlamydia	429.4	387.4	426.0
Gonorrhea	98.5	132.1	100.8

[a]Nationwide estimates are not available for all health indicators in the table
[b]Signifies that no nationwide incidence of the health indicator could be found

Open Access This chapter is distributed under the terms of the Creative Commons Attribution Noncommercial License which permits any noncommercial use, distribution, and reproduction in any medium, provided the original author(s) and source are credited.

References

1. Merriam-Webster Dictionary. 2012. http://www.merriam-webster.com/medical/communica ble%20disease. Accessed May 2012.
2. National Institute of Allergy and Infectious Diseases. Detailed explanation of tuberculosis (TB). 2009. http://1.usa.gov/RFCULq. Accessed May 2012.
3. Pratt R, Price S, Miramontes R, Navin T, Abraham BK. Trends in tuberculosis incidence – United States, 2010. MMWR. 2011;60:333–7.
4. Centers for Disease Control and Prevention. New, simpler way to treat latent TB infection. 2011. http://www.cdc.gov/Features/TuberculosisTreatment. Accessed May 2012.
5. Centers for Disease Control and Prevention. Reported tuberculosis in the United States 2010. Atlanta, GA: U.S. Department of Health and Human Services, Centers for Disease Control and Prevention; 2011.
6. Mayo Clinic Staff. Tuberculosis: risk factors. Mayo Clinic. 2011. http://www.mayoclinic.com/ health/tuberculosis/DS00372/DSECTION=4. Accessed May 2012.
7. National Institute of Allergy and Infectious Diseases. HIV/AIDS. 2011. http://www.niaid.nih. gov/topics/hivaids/understanding/Pages/Default.aspx. Accessed May 2012.
8. Centers for Disease Control and Prevention. Basic information about HIV and AIDS. 2012. http://www.cdc.gov/hiv/topics/basic/. Accessed May 2012.
9. Centers for Disease Control and Prevention. Living with HIV/AIDS. 2007. http://www.cdc. gov/hiv/resources/brochures/livingwithhiv.htm. Accessed May 2012.
10. Mayo Clinic Staff. HIV/AIDS. Mayo Clinic. 2011. http://www.mayoclinic.com/health/hiv-aids/DS00005/. Accessed May 2012.
11. Centers for Disease Control and Prevention. HIV in the United States: at a glance. 2012. http:// www.cdc.gov/hiv/resources/factsheets/us.htm. Accessed May 2012.
12. Centers for Disease Control and Prevention. HIV surveillance report, 2010, vol. 22. 2102. Atlanta, GA: U.S. Department of Health and Human Services. http://www.cdc.gov/hiv/topics/ surveillance/resources/reports/. Accessed May 2012.
13. National Institute of Allergy and Infectious Diseases. Syphilis. 2010. http://www.niaid.nih. gov/topics/syphilis/Pages/default.aspx. Accessed May 2012.

14. Division of STD Prevention. Syphilis – CDC fact sheet. Centers for Disease Control and Prevention. 2010. http://www.cdc.gov/std/syphilis/STDFact-Syphilis.htm. Accessed May 2012.
15. Kamb ML. Congenital syphilis: not gone and all too forgotten. World J Pediatr. 2010; 6:101–2.
16. Centers for Disease Control and Prevention. Sexually transmitted disease surveillance 2010. Atlanta, GA: U.S. Department of Health and Human Services, Centers for Disease Control and Prevention; 2011.
17. Mayo Clinic Staff. Syphilis: risk factors. Mayo Clinic. 2010. http://www.mayoclinic.com/health/syphilis/ds00374/dsection=risk-factors. Accessed May 2012.
18. Division of STD Prevention. Chlamydia – CDC fact sheet. Centers for Disease Control and Prevention. 2012. http://www.cdc.gov/std/chlamydia/STDFact-Chlamydia.htm. Accessed May 2012.
19. National Institute of Allergy and Infectious Diseases. Chlamydia. 2010. http://www.niaid.nih.gov/topics/chlamydia/Pages/default.aspx. Accessed May 2012.
20. Division of STD Prevention. Gonorrhea – CDC fact sheet. Centers for Disease Control and Prevention. 2012. http://www.cdc.gov/std/Gonorrhea/STDFact-gonorrhea.htm. Accessed May 2012.
21. Mayo Clinic Staff. Gonorrhea: risk factors. Mayo Clinic. 2011. http://www.mayoclinic.com/health/gonorrhea/ds00180/dsection=risk-factors. Accessed May 2012.

Chapter 5
Cancer Incidence and Mortality

Cancer is a vital health issue in Texas. Thousands of Texas residents are affected by cancer each year, and cancer is the second leading cause of death in the state and in the nation, accounting for one of every four deaths. More than 1.6 million Americans are expected to be diagnosed with cancer and more than 577,000 Americans are expected to die from cancer-related causes in 2012 [1]. In Texas, more than 110,000 residents are expected to be diagnosed with cancer in 2012, and more than 39,000 cancer-related deaths are expected [2].

Cancer begins when certain cells in the body change and start to grow abnormally and uncontrollably. Cancer cells can also invade other organs and tissues and be spread by the bloodstream and lymphatic system in a process called metastasis. This uncontrolled growth and spread of cancer can result in serious health problems and death. Currently, doctors cannot determine what causes cancer in an individual person, but there are several risk factors that may play a role in cancer development including aging, tobacco, alcohol consumption, sunlight, ionizing radiation, certain viruses and bacteria, poor nutrition, lack of physical activity, being overweight, certain hormones, and certain chemicals [3]. Many of these risk factors can be avoided, thus lowering a person's risk of developing cancer. Other risk factors cannot be avoided, but many cancers can be cured if detected and treated early. Incidence and mortality rates for each cancer are presented as age-adjusted rates or age-specific rates.

Breast Cancer

Breast cancer usually develops in cells that line the ducts that carry milk to the nipples (ductal cancer) or in cells of the glands, which make milk (lobular cancer). Ductal cancer is more common than lobular cancer. Although more rare, cancer can also occur in other tissues of the breast [4]. Breast cancer is the most common diagnosis of cancer in Texas and US women [1]. It is estimated that in 2012,

A.G. Ramirez et al. (eds.), *The South Texas Health Status Review:*
A Health Disparities Roadmap, DOI 10.1007/978-3-319-00233-0_5, © The Author(s) 2013

approximately 16,127 Texas women will be diagnosed
with invasive breast cancer and 2,867 women will die of
the disease [2]. Breast cancer occurs most frequently in
women, but men can also develop breast cancer. Hispanic
women have a lower risk of developing breast cancer
than non-Hispanic women, who are at greater risk than
African-American women [5].

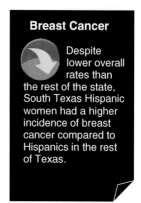

Breast Cancer

Despite lower overall rates than the rest of the state, South Texas Hispanic women had a higher incidence of breast cancer compared to Hispanics in the rest of Texas.

Increasing age is the most important risk factor for
breast cancer [1, 6]. Other risk factors include a personal or family history of breast cancer, genetic muta-
tions in the BRCA1 or BRCA2 genes, certain breast
changes such as atypical hyperplasia, high breast tissue
density, high dose radiation to the chest, and certain
reproductive factors such as never having children, having a first child after age
30, or having menstrual periods start early or end late in life. Modifiable risk factors for breast cancer include lack of physical activity, alcohol use, being overweight after menopause, and oral contraceptive use [1, 7]. Screening tests for
breast cancer include the breast self-exam, clinical breast exam, and screening
mammography [7].

Breast Cancer in South Texas

Overall, women in South Texas had a lower average annual age-adjusted incidence
of breast cancer (106.3 cases per 100,000 women) than women in the rest of Texas
(117.5/100,000) or nation (124.0/100,000). However, Hispanic women in South
Texas had a higher incidence of breast cancer (95.6/100,000) than Hispanics in the
rest of Texas (90.7/100,000), although they did not have a statistically significantly
higher breast cancer incidence compared to Hispanic women nationwide (Fig. 5.1).
Hispanic women overall, including those in South Texas, had a much lower
incidence of breast cancer than non-Hispanic white women (Fig. 5.1).

Similar age trends for breast cancer incidence were seen for both Hispanic and
non-Hispanic white women in South Texas. Similar to what was observed in the rest
of Texas, the risk of breast cancer in South Texas generally increased with age.
Among women aged 45 and older, the incidence of breast cancer in non-Hispanic
whites was higher than in Hispanics (Fig. 5.2).

In 2005–2009, a higher average annual age-adjusted incidence of breast cancer
was seen in South Texas metropolitan counties (107.7/100,000) than nonmetropolitan counties (97.2/100,000). Overall, Bexar County had a higher incidence of breast
cancer (117.2/100,000) than South Texas as a whole (106.3/100,000), and the Lower
Rio Grande Valley area had a lower breast cancer incidence (90.6/100,000) compared to South Texas overall (Fig. 5.3).

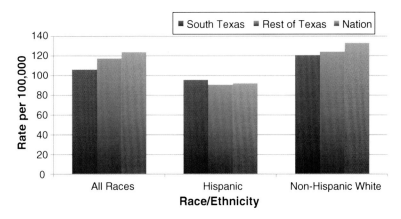

Fig. 5.1 Age-adjusted incidence of breast cancer in females by location. *Sources*: Texas incidence: Texas Cancer Registry, Cancer Epidemiology and Surveillance Branch, Texas Department of State Health Services, 2005–2009 data; Nationwide incidence: National Cancer Institute, 17-region SEER data, 2004–2008

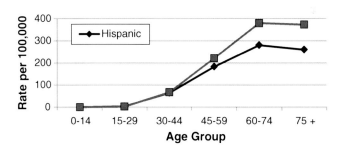

Fig. 5.2 Incidence of breast cancer in South Texas females by age group and race/ethnicity, 2005–2009. *Source*: Texas Cancer Registry, Cancer Epidemiology and Surveillance Branch, Texas Department of State Health Services

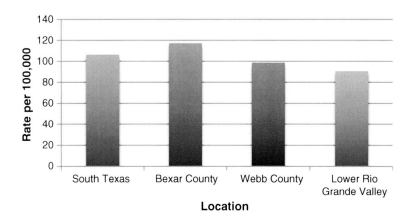

Fig. 5.3 Age-adjusted incidence of female breast cancer in selected South Texas locations, 2005–2009. *Source*: Texas Cancer Registry, Cancer Epidemiology and Surveillance Branch, Texas Department of State Health Services

The overall breast cancer mortality rate among females in South Texas was 19.7/100,000. For the most part, breast cancer mortality rate patterns in South Texas were similar to incidence patterns.

Cervical Cancer

Cervical cancer typically begins in the lining of the cervix, which is the lower section of the uterus and connects the upper section of the uterus to the vagina. There are two main types of cervical cancer. By far, the most common type is squamous cell carcinoma, which develops from the cells that line the outer surface of the cervix near the top of the vagina. The other type is adenocarcinoma, which develops from the glandular cells that line the cervix [8]. There are usually no symptoms of precancerous changes to the cervix. Therefore, regular screening tests such as Pap tests, which can detect abnormal cervical cells before cancer develops, are of great importance [8, 9].

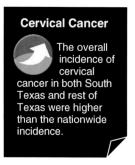

Cervical Cancer

The overall incidence of cervical cancer in both South Texas and rest of Texas were higher than the nationwide incidence.

Even though cervical cancer is one of the most detectable and preventable cancers through regular screening, it remains a serious threat to the lives of Texas women. In 2012, an estimated 1,255 Texas women will be diagnosed with invasive cervical cancer and 392 women will die of the disease [10]. In the USA, Hispanic women are at greater risk of developing cervical cancer than non-Hispanic white women, and African-American women are at greater risk of cervical cancer than are non-Hispanic white women [5].

Certain human papillomaviruses (HPVs) are the most important risk factors for cervical cancer [8, 9]. An HPV vaccine is currently available for girls and women aged 9–26 that may help protect against as much as 70 % of cervical cancer [11, 12]. Women with HIV or other conditions that result in a weakened immune system are also at higher risk of cervical cancer. Other modifiable risk factors include smoking, sexual history, and long-term use of oral contraceptives [8].

Cervical Cancer in South Texas

Overall, cervical cancer incidence was higher among women in South Texas (10.5 cases per 100,000 women) than in the rest of Texas (9.3/100,000) in 2005–2009 (Fig. 5.4). The overall incidence of cervical cancer in both South Texas and rest of Texas were higher than the nationwide incidence (8.1/100,000). As in the rest of Texas and nationwide, Hispanic women in South Texas had a higher incidence of cervical cancer than non-Hispanic whites (Fig. 5.4). This ethnic difference in incidence was not as large in South Texas as in the rest of Texas, however.

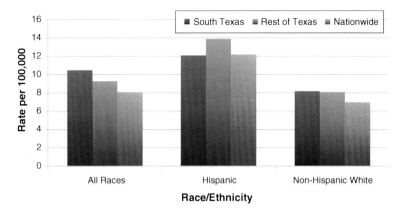

Fig. 5.4 Age-adjusted incidence of cervical cancer in females by location. *Sources*: Texas incidence: Texas Cancer Registry, Cancer Epidemiology and Surveillance Branch, Texas Department of State Health Services, 2005–2009 data; Nationwide incidence: National Cancer Institute, 17-region SEER data, 2004–2008

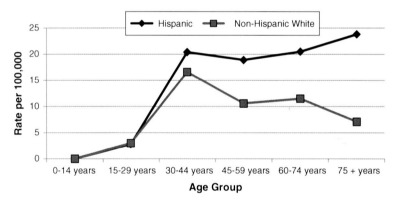

Fig. 5.5 Incidence of cervical cancer in South Texas females by age group, 2005–2009. *Source*: Texas Cancer Registry, Cancer Epidemiology and Surveillance Branch, Texas Department of State Health Services

In South Texas, as in the rest of Texas, age-specific trends in cervical cancer incidence differed between Hispanics and non-Hispanic whites. Incidence peaked in non-Hispanic white women at ages 30–44 but continued to rise with age in Hispanic women (Fig. 5.5). This observation is of particular concern for Hispanics because research suggests that women diagnosed with cervical cancer at ages 50 or older are more likely than younger women to have an advanced stage of the disease [13]. The incidence of cervical cancer in Hispanics was significantly higher than in non-Hispanic whites for ages 45 and older (Fig. 5.5).

The overall cervical cancer mortality rate among females in South Texas was 3.4/100,000. Cervical cancer mortality rate patterns were similar to those for cervical cancer incidence.

Colorectal Cancer

Colorectal cancer begins either in the colon (the first 4–5 feet of the large intestine) or the rectum (the last few inches of the large intestine before the anus) [14]. Colorectal cancer is generally slow to develop and usually begins in a noncancerous polyp, which can be removed during a colonoscopy, thus preventing invasive colorectal cancer. The most common type of colorectal cancer is adenocarcinoma, a cancer that begins in glandular tissue in the internal lining of the colon or rectum [15]. Screening tests include the fecal occult blood test, sigmoidoscopy, colonoscopy, double contrast barium enema, and digital rectal exam [16].

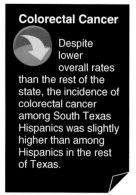

Colorectal Cancer

Despite lower overall rates than the rest of the state, the incidence of colorectal cancer among South Texas Hispanics was slightly higher than among Hispanics in the rest of Texas.

Colorectal cancer is the third-most common cancer diagnosis and cause of cancer death in both men and women in the USA and Texas [17]. In 2012, an estimated 10,604 Texas residents will be diagnosed with colorectal cancer and 3,721 will die of the disease [2]. In the USA, men have a higher risk of colorectal cancer than women [17]. Hispanics are at lower risk of developing colorectal cancer than non-Hispanic whites, and African-Americans are at greater risk than non-Hispanic whites [17]. Incidence of colorectal cancer increases with age. In the USA, more than 90 % of all colorectal cancers are diagnosed in those aged 50 or older [17].

Risk factors for colorectal cancer include having colorectal polyps, a personal or family history of colorectal cancer, or certain diseases that cause inflammation of the large intestine such as Crohn's disease or ulcerative colitis. Modifiable risk factors include obesity, lack of physical activity, diet (a high intake of red or processed meat and a low intake of fruits and vegetables), smoking, and heavy alcohol consumption [16, 17].

Colorectal Cancer in South Texas

Colorectal cancer incidence was lower in South Texas (41.7 cases per 100,000 population) than in the rest of Texas (44.8/100,000) or nation (47.2/100,000). However, the incidence of colorectal cancer among Hispanics in South Texas was slightly higher than the incidence among Hispanics in the rest of Texas (Fig. 5.6).

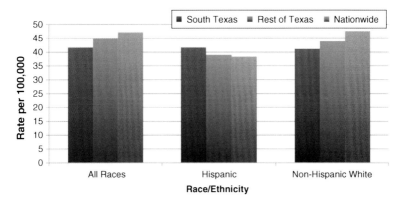

Fig. 5.6 Age-adjusted incidence of colorectal cancer by location. *Sources*: Texas incidence: Texas Cancer Registry, Cancer Epidemiology and Surveillance Branch, Texas Department of State Health Services, 2005–2009 data; Nationwide incidence: National Cancer Institute, 17-region SEER data, 2004–2008

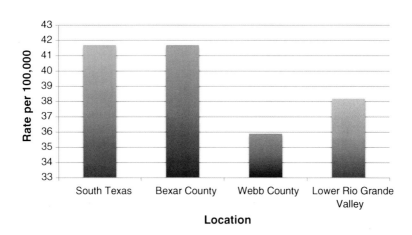

Fig. 5.7 Age-adjusted incidence of colorectal cancer in selected South Texas locations, 2005–2009. *Source*: Texas Cancer Registry, Cancer Epidemiology and Surveillance Branch, Texas Department of State Health Services

In South Texas, non-Hispanic whites and Hispanics were diagnosed with colorectal cancer at similar rates in 2005–2009 (Fig. 5.6).

Sex and age patterns of colorectal cancer incidence were the same in South Texas as observed nationwide. In South Texas, males had a much higher incidence of colorectal cancer (52.5/100,000) than females (33.0/100,000), and the risk of colorectal cancer increased with age.

Webb County and the Lower Rio Grande Valley region both had lower incidence rates of colorectal cancer than all of South Texas (Fig. 5.7).

The overall colorectal cancer mortality rate in South Texas was 13.9/100,000. Unlike incidence, colorectal cancer mortality rates among Hispanics in South Texas and the rest of Texas were very similar. For all other comparisons, colorectal cancer mortality rate patterns were similar to those for colorectal cancer incidence.

Prostate Cancer

Prostate cancer develops in the prostate gland, which is a male reproductive system gland located beneath the bladder, in front of the rectum, and surrounding the urethra. The prostate gland makes some of the fluid in semen [18, 19]. Prostate cancer is generally very slow to grow, and many men will develop prostate cancer if they reach advanced age [18]. Screening tests include the digital rectal exam and the blood test for prostate-specific antigen (PSA test) [19].

Prostate Cancer

Despite overall rates than the rest of the state, Hispanics in Webb County and the Lower Rio Grande Valley region had significantly higher incidence rates of prostate cancer than Hispanics in South Texas overall.

Prostate cancer is the most common cancer diagnosis and the second leading cause of cancer death in men, both in Texas and nationwide [1]. In 2012, an estimated 16,777 Texas men will be diagnosed with invasive prostate cancer and 1,779 will die of the disease [2]. Hispanic men are at lower risk of developing colorectal cancer than non-Hispanics, and African-American men are at greater risk than whites. The risk of prostate cancer increases with age. Besides age and race/ethnicity, the only other well-known risk factor for prostate cancer is a family history of the disease [1, 19].

Prostate Cancer Incidence in South Texas

Prostate cancer incidence in South Texas (121.2 cases per 100,000 men) was lower than in the rest of Texas (146.4/100,000) and nation (156.0/100,000) (Fig. 5.8). As observed in the rest of Texas and nationwide, non-Hispanic white men in South Texas had a higher incidence of prostate cancer than Hispanic men (Fig. 5.8).

Prostate cancer incidence increased with age for both Hispanic and non-Hispanic white men in South Texas up to ages 70–74. However, at ages 75 and older, incidence declined among whites and leveled off a bit among Hispanics (Fig. 5.9). Non-Hispanic white men had a higher risk of prostate cancer than Hispanic men aged 30–74.

In South Texas, the incidence of prostate cancer among men living in metropolitan counties (121.0/100,000) was very similar to the incidence among those in nonmetropolitan counties (120.8/100,000). Overall, the incidence of prostate cancer in Bexar County, Webb County, and the Lower Rio Grande Valley region were all

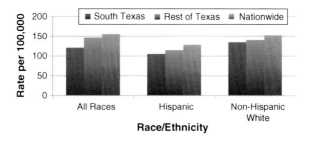

Fig. 5.8 Age-adjusted incidence of prostate cancer among males, by location. *Sources*: Texas incidence: Texas Cancer Registry, Cancer Epidemiology and Surveillance Branch, Texas Department of State Health Services, 2005–2009 data; Nationwide incidence: National Cancer Institute, 17-region SEER data, 2004–2008

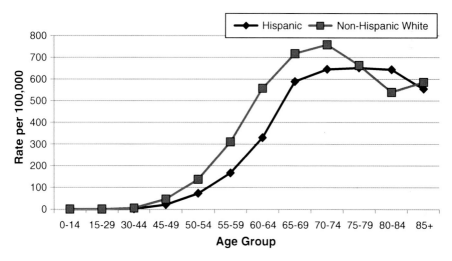

Fig. 5.9 Incidence of prostate cancer among South Texas males, by age group and race/ethnicity, 2005–2009. *Source*: Texas Cancer Registry, Cancer Epidemiology and Surveillance Branch, Texas Department of State Health Services

similar to the incidence in South Texas as a whole. However, Hispanics in Webb County and the Lower Rio Grande Valley region had significantly higher incidence rates of prostate cancer than Hispanics in South Texas overall, while Hispanics in Bexar County had a significantly lower rate of prostate cancer than in South Texas overall (Fig. 5.10).

The overall prostate cancer mortality rate in South Texas was 18.8/100,000. Like incidence, prostate cancer mortality rates were lower in South Texas than in the rest of Texas or nation. No significant differences in prostate cancer mortality rates were seen between Hispanic and non-Hispanic white men in South Texas, nor between South Texas Hispanic and non-Hispanic white men when compared to Hispanics and non-Hispanic white men in the rest of Texas (Fig. 5.11).

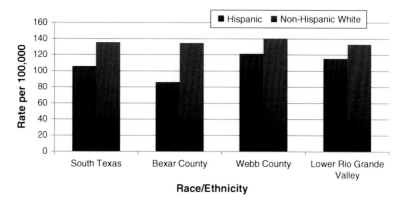

Fig. 5.10 Age-adjusted incidence of prostate cancer among South Texas males in selected South Texas locations, by race/ethnicity, 2005–2009. *Source*: Texas Cancer Registry, Cancer Epidemiology and Surveillance Branch, Texas Department of State Health Services

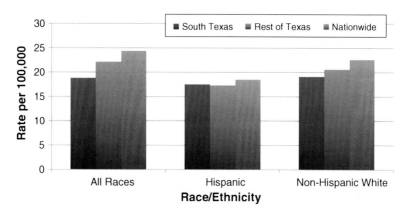

Fig. 5.11 Age-adjusted mortality rate of prostate cancer among males, by location. *Sources*: Texas mortality: Texas Cancer Registry, Cancer Epidemiology and Surveillance Branch, Texas Department of State Health Services, 2005–2009 data; Nationwide mortality: National Cancer Institute, 17-region SEER data, 2004–2008

The trend in age-specific prostate cancer mortality for South Texas was different from the trend seen in prostate cancer incidence; mortality rates continued to increase among the oldest age groups (Fig. 5.12).

Lung and Bronchus Cancer

Lung and bronchus cancers are cancers of the respiratory system. The bronchi are tubes that connect the trachea (windpipe) with smaller tubes in the lungs called bronchioles [20, 21]. Most lung cancers not only begin in cells that line the bronchi

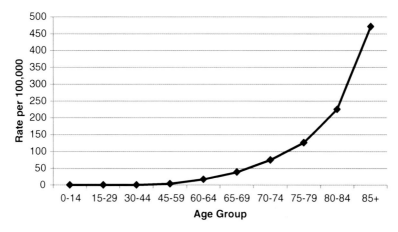

Fig. 5.12 Prostate cancer mortality among South Texas males by age group, 2005–2009. *Source*: Texas Cancer Registry, Cancer Epidemiology and Surveillance Branch, Texas Department of State Health Services

but also can begin in other parts of the lung such as the bronchioles or alveoli (tiny air sacs attached to the bronchioles) [21].

For treatment purposes, lung and bronchus cancer are grouped into small cell cancers and nonsmall cell cancers, which account for 10–15 % and 85–90 % of all lung and bronchus cancers, respectively [21, 22]. Small cell lung cancer grows more quickly than nonsmall cell lung cancer and is more likely to metastasize; however, it is less common than nonsmall cell lung cancer [22]. There are no recommended screening tests for lung and bronchus cancer for asymptomatic people [1].

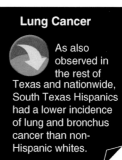

Lung Cancer

As also observed in the rest of Texas and nationwide, South Texas Hispanics had a lower incidence of lung and bronchus cancer than non-Hispanic whites.

Lung and bronchus cancer is the second-most common cancer diagnosis and the leading cause of cancer death among both men and women in the USA and Texas [1]. In 2012, an estimated 14,555 Texans will be diagnosed with lung and bronchus cancer and 10,608 will die of the disease [23]. In the USA, males have a higher risk of lung and bronchus cancer than females [1]. Hispanic men and women are at lower risk of developing lung and bronchus cancer than non-Hispanics. African-American men are at greater risk of lung and bronchus cancer than white men, while white women have a higher risk than African-American women [5]. The most important risk factor for lung and bronchus cancer is cigarette smoking [1]. Other risk factors include exposure to secondhand cigarette smoke, radon, asbestos, certain metals, certain organic chemicals, and air pollution [1, 20].

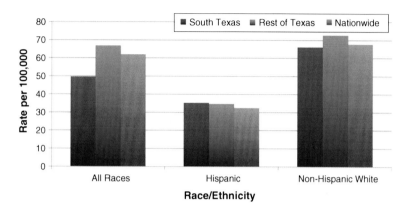

Fig. 5.13 Age-adjusted incidence of lung and bronchus cancer by location. *Sources*: Texas incidence: Texas Cancer Registry, Cancer Epidemiology and Surveillance Branch, Texas Department of State Health Services, 2005–2009 data; Nationwide incidence: National Cancer Institute, 17-region SEER data, 2004–2008

Lung and Bronchus Cancer in South Texas

The incidence of lung and bronchus cancer in South Texas in 2005–2009 (49.6 cases per 100,000 population) was lower than the rest of Texas (66.9/100,000) and nation (62.0/100,000). Hispanics in South Texas had a similar incidence of lung and bronchus cancer as Hispanics in the rest of Texas; however, non-Hispanic whites in South Texas had a lower incidence (66.1/100,000) than non-Hispanic whites in the rest of Texas (72.8/100,000). As also observed in the rest of Texas and nationwide, Hispanics in South Texas had a lower incidence of lung and bronchus cancer than non-Hispanic whites, who had almost twice the risk of lung cancer as Hispanics (Fig. 5.13).

The incidence of lung and bronchus cancer is very rare until ages 30–44 and then rises until ages 75–79 for non-Hispanic whites and ages 80–84 for Hispanics (Fig. 5.14). Among those aged 45 and older in South Texas, non-Hispanic whites have a statistically significantly higher lung and bronchus cancer incidence than Hispanics.

As seen nationwide, South Texas males had a higher incidence of lung and bronchus cancer than females. The incidence of lung and bronchus cancer was 1.7 times higher among non-Hispanic white males than non-Hispanic white females and was 2.4 times higher among Hispanic males than Hispanic females (Fig. 5.15).

The lung and bronchus cancer mortality rate in South Texas was 36.2/100,000. For the most part, lung cancer mortality rate patterns were similar to those for lung cancer incidence.

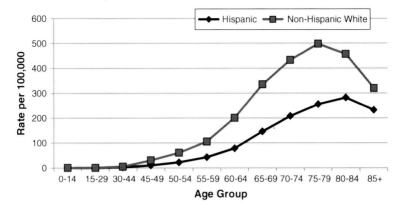

Fig. 5.14 Incidence of lung and bronchus cancer in South Texas by age group and race/ethnicity, 2005–2009. *Source*: Texas Cancer Registry, Cancer Epidemiology and Surveillance Branch, Texas Department of State Health Services

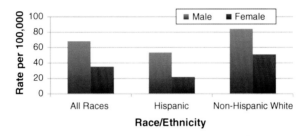

Fig. 5.15 Age-adjusted incidence of lung and bronchus cancer in South Texas by sex and race/ethnicity, 2005–2009. *Source*: Texas Cancer Registry, Cancer Epidemiology and Surveillance Branch, Texas Department of State Health Services

Liver and Intrahepatic Bile Duct Cancer

Liver and intrahepatic bile duct cancer occurs either in the liver, an organ that metabolizes nutrients, makes bile, and detoxifies chemicals, or in intrahepatic bile ducts, tubes within the liver that carry bile to the gallbladder. There are no recommended screening tests for liver and intrahepatic bile duct cancer for asymptomatic people [24].

Liver and intrahepatic bile duct cancer is relatively rare in the USA and in Texas. In 2012, an estimated 2,197 Texas residents will be diagnosed with liver and intrahepatic bile duct cancer and 1,768 residents will die of the disease [25]. The incidence of liver and

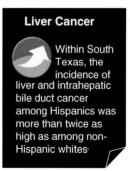

Liver Cancer

Within South Texas, the incidence of liver and intrahepatic bile duct cancer among Hispanics was more than twice as high as among non-Hispanic whites·

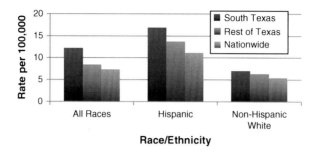

Fig. 5.16 Age-adjusted incidence of liver and intrahepatic bile duct cancer by location. *Sources*: Texas incidence: Texas Cancer Registry, Cancer Epidemiology and Surveillance Branch, Texas Department of State Health Services, 2005–2009 data; Nationwide incidence: National Cancer Institute, 17-region SEER data, 2004–2008

intrahepatic bile duct cancer increases with age, and men are twice as likely as women to develop liver cancer [26]. Hispanic men and women have a much higher risk of developing liver and intrahepatic bile duct cancer than non-Hispanics. Risk factors for liver and intrahepatic bile duct cancer include heavy alcohol use, chronic infection with hepatitis B or hepatitis C, and family history of liver cancer [24, 26].

Liver and Intrahepatic Bile Duct Cancer in South Texas

The South Texas incidence of liver and intrahepatic bile duct cancer was 12.2 cases per 100,000 population in 2005–2009, about a 50 % higher incidence than in the rest of Texas (8.4/100,000) and nation (7.3/100,000) (Fig. 5.16). In South Texas, the incidence of liver and intrahepatic bile duct cancer among Hispanics was more than twice as high as that among non-Hispanic whites (rate ratio = 2.4) (Fig. 5.16).

The incidence of liver and intrahepatic bile duct cancer was more than three times greater in South Texas males than in females (19.5/100,000 vs. 6.2/100,000). As observed nationwide, liver and intrahepatic bile duct cancer incidence in South Texas increased with age. The incidence of liver cancer was very low until ages 45–49. Among older age groups (ages 55 and older), Hispanics had a significantly higher rate of liver and intrahepatic bile duct cancer than non-Hispanic whites, and this rate differential increased with increasing age (Fig. 5.17).

In South Texas, the incidence of liver and intrahepatic bile duct cancer was slightly but not significantly higher in metropolitan counties (12.5/100,000) than nonmetropolitan counties (10.8/100,000). Liver and intrahepatic bile duct cancer incidence in the Lower Rio Grande Valley region (11.8/100,000) was similar to the incidence for South Texas as a whole (12.2/100,000). Rates for Webb and Bexar counties were slightly higher than those in South Texas as a whole, but only Bexar County's incidence rate was statistically significant (Fig. 5.18).

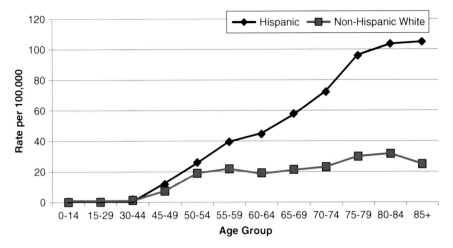

Fig. 5.17 Incidence of liver and intrahepatic bile duct cancer in South Texas by age group and race/ethnicity, 2005–2009. *Source*: Texas Cancer Registry, Cancer Epidemiology and Surveillance Branch, Texas Department of State Health Services

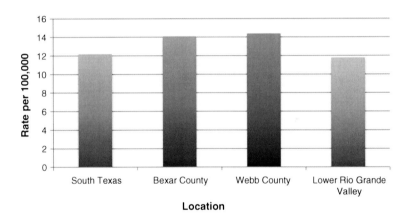

Fig. 5.18 Age-adjusted incidence of liver and intrahepatic bile duct cancer in selected *South Texas locations, 2005–2009. Source*: Texas Cancer Registry, Cancer Epidemiology and Surveillance Branch, Texas Department of State Health Services

The overall liver and intrahepatic bile duct cancer mortality rate in South Texas was 9.3/100,000. For the most part, patterns of liver cancer mortality rate in South Texas were similar to those for liver cancer incidence.

Stomach Cancer

Stomach cancer, also called gastric cancer, usually develops in the cells that line the inside of the stomach. There are no recommended screening tests for stomach cancer in asymptomatic people [27].

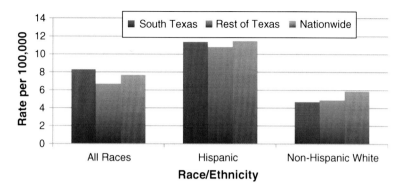

Fig. 5.19 Age-adjusted incidence of stomach cancer by location, 2005–2009. *Sources*: Texas incidence: Texas Cancer Registry, Cancer Epidemiology and Surveillance Branch, Texas Department of State Health Services, 2005–2009 data; Nationwide incidence: National Cancer Institute, 17-region SEER data, 2004–2008

Stomach cancer is a relatively rare cancer both in the USA and in Texas. In 2012, an estimated 1,731 Texas residents will be diagnosed with stomach cancer and 954 will die of the disease [25]. The US average annual age-adjusted incidence rate of stomach cancer for 2004–2008 was 10.8 cases per 100,000 in men and 5.4/100,000 in women. Hispanic men and women have a higher risk of developing stomach cancer than non-Hispanics whites [27]. The incidence of stomach cancer increases with age. Other risk factors for stomach cancer include *Helicobacter pylori* infection, certain health conditions such as pernicious anemia or chronic gastritis, and a family history of stomach cancer. Modifiable risk factors include smoking and a diet high in smoked, salted, or pickled foods [28].

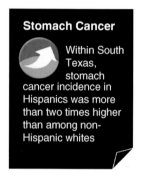

Stomach Cancer

Within South Texas, stomach cancer incidence in Hispanics was more than two times higher than among non-Hispanic whites

Stomach Cancer in South Texas

South Texas had a slightly higher incidence of stomach cancer (8.3/100,000) than the rest of Texas (6.7/100,000) or nation (7.7/100,000). In South Texas, stomach cancer incidence in Hispanics (11.4/100,000) was more than two times higher than the incidence in non-Hispanic whites (4.7/100,000) (Fig. 5.19).

As observed nationwide, the incidence of stomach cancer in South Texas residents increased with age. Hispanics had a higher stomach cancer incidence than non-Hispanic whites among persons aged 45 and older (Fig. 5.20).

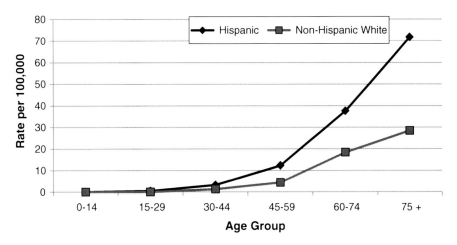

Fig. 5.20 Incidence of stomach cancer in South Texas by age group and race/ethnicity, 2005–2009. *Source*: Texas Cancer Registry, Cancer Epidemiology and Surveillance Branch, Texas Department of State Health Services

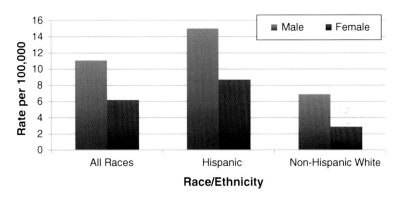

Fig. 5.21 Age-adjusted incidence of stomach cancer in South Texas by sex and race/ethnicity, 2005–2009. *Source*: Texas Cancer Registry, Cancer Epidemiology and Surveillance Branch, Texas Department of State Health Services

In South Texas, the incidence of stomach cancer was almost two times higher in Hispanic males than in Hispanic females, and stomach cancer incidence was 2.4 times higher in non-Hispanic white males than in non-Hispanic white females (Fig. 5.21).

The overall stomach cancer mortality rate in South Texas was 4.6/100,000. Stomach cancer mortality rate patterns were similar to those for stomach cancer incidence.

Gallbladder Cancer

Gallbladder cancer usually develops in cells that line the inside of the gallbladder, a small pear-shaped organ that stores bile and is located below the right lobe of the liver [29].

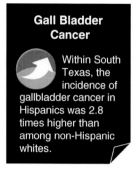

Gall Bladder Cancer

Within South Texas, the incidence of gallbladder cancer in Hispanics was 2.8 times higher than among non-Hispanic whites.

Gallbladder cancer is a relatively rare cancer in both the USA and in Texas. In 2012, an estimated 9,810 new cases of gallbladder and other biliary cancer are expected in the USA as well as 3,200 deaths [1]. In the USA, gallbladder cancer is most common in Hispanic and Native American populations. Women are more than twice as likely as men to develop gallbladder cancer. Incidence of gallbladder cancer increases with age; three of every four people diagnosed with gallbladder cancer in the USA are older than age 65 [29]. Other risk factors for gallbladder cancer include having gallstones and inflammation of the gallbladder, typhoid, a family history of gallbladder cancer, and exposure to certain industrial chemicals. Obesity is a modifiable risk factor for gallbladder cancer [29].

Gallbladder Cancer in South Texas

Overall, South Texas had a higher incidence of gallbladder cancer (1.7 cases per 100,000 population) than the rest of Texas (1.1/100,000) and nation (1.2/100,000). In South Texas, the incidence of gallbladder cancer in Hispanics (2.5/100,000) was 2.8 times higher than the incidence in non-Hispanic whites (0.9/100,000) (Fig. 5.22).

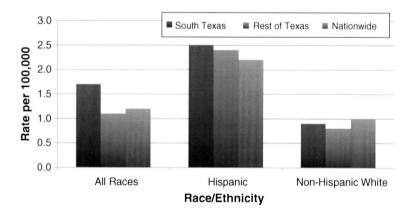

Fig. 5.22 Age-adjusted incidence of gallbladder cancer by location. *Sources*: Texas incidence: Texas Cancer Registry, Cancer Epidemiology and Surveillance Branch, Texas Department of State Health Services, 2005–2009 data; Nationwide incidence: National Cancer Institute, 17-region SEER data, 2004–2008

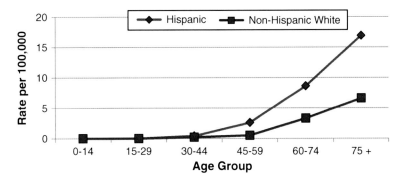

Fig. 5.23 Incidence of gallbladder cancer in South Texas by age group and race/ethnicity, 2005–2009. *Source*: Texas Cancer Registry, Cancer Epidemiology and Surveillance Branch, Texas Department of State Health Services

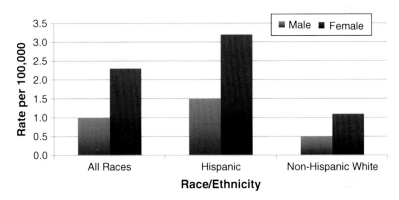

Fig. 5.24 Age-adjusted incidence of gallbladder cancer in South Texas by sex and race/ethnicity, 2005–2009. *Source*: Texas Cancer Registry, Cancer Epidemiology and Surveillance Branch, Texas Department of State Health Services

As observed nationwide, the incidence of gallbladder cancer in South Texas increased with age. The difference in gallbladder cancer incidence between Hispanics and non-Hispanic whites grew with age, too (Fig. 5.23), and Hispanics aged 45 and older had a significantly higher incidence of gallbladder cancer than non-Hispanic whites.

In South Texas, gallbladder cancer incidence was higher in females (2.3/100,000) than males (1.0/100,000). Among both Hispanics and non-Hispanic whites in South Texas, females had roughly twice the risk of gallbladder cancer as males (Fig. 5.24).

The overall gallbladder cancer mortality rate in South Texas was 0.8/100,000. Gallbladder cancer mortality rate patterns were similar to those for gallbladder cancer incidence.

Childhood and Adolescent Leukemia

Leukemia is a cancer that develops in bone marrow in cells that eventually circulate in the blood or lymphatic system. Leukemia can be classified by the type of cell where lymphocytes (a type of white blood cell) and is called lymphocytic leukemia. Leukemias that start in other types of immature cells found in the blood, such as red blood cells, white blood cells other than lymphocytes, and platelets, are called myelogenous (or myeloid) leukemias. Leukemias can also be divided into two additional groups, chronic or acute. Most leukemia in children is acute [30].

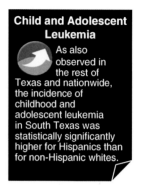

Child and Adolescent Leukemia

As also observed in the rest of Texas and nationwide, the incidence of childhood and adolescent leukemia in South Texas was statistically significantly higher for Hispanics than for non-Hispanic whites.

Leukemia is the most common cancer in children and adolescents, both in the USA and in Texas [30]. Roughly one-third of all childhood cancers are leukemias [1]. Among children with leukemia, about 75 % will be diagnosed with acute lymphocytic leukemia (ALL) [1, 30]. Most of the remaining cases of childhood leukemia will be acute myelogenous leukemia (AML). There are no recommended screening tests for leukemia in asymptomatic children or adolescents [30].

Cancer in children and adolescents is relatively rare. Over 10 years (2000–2009), there were 2,859 cases of leukemia, myeloproliferative or myelodysplastic disease in Texas children aged 0–14, and an additional 548 cases in adolescents aged 15–19 [31]. Hispanic children and adolescents are at slightly higher risk of developing leukemia, myeloproliferative or myelodysplastic disease compared to non-Hispanic white children and adolescents, while African-American children and adolescents have the lowest risk [5].In general, rates of leukemia, myeloproliferative or myelodysplastic disease are slightly higher in boys than girls [5, 30]. Little is known about the risk factors for childhood and adolescent leukemia. The few known risk factors include radiation exposure and certain genetic conditions such as Down's syndrome and Li–Fraumeni syndrome [30].

Childhood and Adolescent Leukemia in South Texas

Overall, the incidence of childhood and adolescent leukemia in South Texas from 2000 to 2009 (53.5 cases per million children or adolescents) was higher than the incidence in the rest of Texas (46.0/million) or nation (44.9/million). However, Hispanics and non-Hispanic whites in South Texas had fairly similar incidences of childhood and adolescent leukemia compared to their counterparts in the rest of Texas and nationwide (Fig. 5.25). As also observed in the rest of Texas and nationwide, the incidence of childhood and adolescent leukemia in South Texas was statistically significantly higher for Hispanics (58.1/million) than for non-Hispanic whites (40.7/million) (Fig. 5.25).

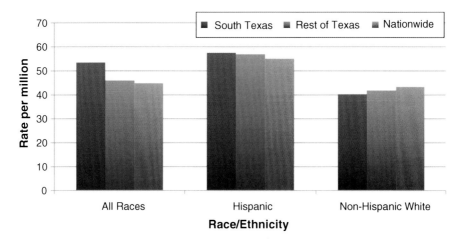

Fig. 5.25 Age-adjusted incidence of child and adolescent leukemia by location, 2000–2009. *Sources*: Texas incidence: Texas Cancer Registry, Cancer Epidemiology and Surveillance Branch, Texas Department of State Health Services, 2000–2009 data; Nationwide incidence: National Cancer Institute, 17-region SEER data, 1999–2008

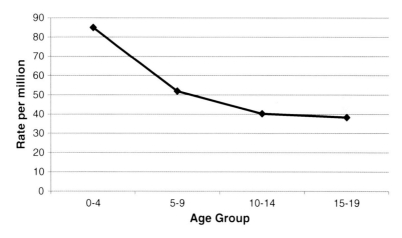

Fig. 5.26 Incidence of child and adolescent leukemia in South Texas by age group, 2000–2009. *Source*: Texas Cancer Registry, Cancer Epidemiology and Surveillance Branch, Texas Department of State Health Services

In South Texas, the incidence of childhood leukemia (58.6/million) was about one-and-a-half times higher than the incidence of adolescent leukemia (38.3/million) during 2000–2009. As is true both statewide and nationally, the incidence of leukemia in South Texas decreased with age. Incidence was highest among children aged 0–4 (Fig. 5.26) [32, 33].

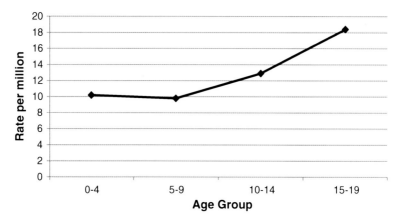

Fig. 5.27 Child and adolescent leukemia mortality in South Texas by age group, 2000–2009. *Source*: Texas Cancer Registry, Cancer Epidemiology and Surveillance Branch, Texas Department of State Health Services

As observed nationwide, incidence of childhood and adolescent leukemia in South Texas was higher for males (62.8/million) than females (43.7/million). The overall child and adolescent leukemia mortality rate in South Texas was 12.8/million. The trend in age-specific child and adolescent leukemia was quite different than the trend in incidence; the highest mortality rate was seen among the adolescent (15–19) age group (Fig. 5.27). This is also true statewide and nationally; leukemia subtypes differ with age at diagnosis, resulting in less favorable survival rates for infants less than 1 year, followed by adolescents aged 15–19 [33].

Summary: Cancer Incidence and Mortality

Table 5.1 Summary table of age-adjusted incidence in South Texas, the rest of Texas, and nationwide for each of the cancer types analyzed

Cancer type	Incidence per 100,000 population[a]		
	South Texas, 2005–2009	Rest of Texas, 2005–2009	USA, 2004–2008
Breast cancer	106.3	117.5	124.0
Cervical cancer	10.5	9.3	8.1
Colorectal cancer	41.7	44.8	47.2
Prostate cancer	121.2	146.4	156.0
Lung and bronchus cancer	49.6	66.9	62.0
Liver and intrahepatic bile duct cancer	12.2	8.4	7.3
Stomach cancer	8.3	6.7	7.7
Gallbladder cancer	1.7	1.1	1.2
Childhood and adolescent leukemia (2000–2009)	53.5 per million	46.0 per million	44.9 per million

[a]All rates except child and adolescent leukemia are expressed in terms of incidence per 100,000 population. Child and adolescent leukemia, however, is expressed in terms of incidence per million population

Table 5.2 Summary table of age-adjusted mortality rates in South Texas, the rest of Texas, and nationwide for each of the cancer types analyzed

Cancer type	Mortality per 100,000 population[a]		
	South Texas, 2005–2009	Rest of Texas, 2005–2009	USA, 2004–2008
Breast cancer	19.7	22.7	23.5
Cervical cancer	3.4	2.8	2.4
Colorectal cancer	13.9	16.7	17.1
Prostate cancer	18.8	22.1	24.4
Lung and bronchus cancer	36.2	50.2	51.6
Liver and intrahepatic bile duct cancer	9.3	6.7	5.3
Stomach cancer	4.6	3.7	3.7
Gallbladder cancer	0.8	0.6	0.6
Childhood and adolescent leukemia (2000–2009)	12.0 per million	7.7 per million	8.0 per million

[a]All rates except child and adolescent leukemia are expressed in terms of mortality per 100,000 population. Child and adolescent leukemia is expressed in terms of mortality per million population

References

1. American Cancer Society. Cancer facts and figures 2012. Atlanta, GA: American Cancer Society; 2012.
2. Texas Department of State Health Services. Texas cancer registry. Expected new cancer cases and deaths by primary site, Texas, 2012. 2012. http://www.dshs.state.tx.us/Expected-Numbers-of-Cancer-Cases-and-Deaths-Texas-2012.aspx. Accessed Feb 2012.
3. National Cancer Institute. What you need to know about cancer – an overview: risk factors. 2006. http://www.cancer.gov/cancertopics/wyntk/cancer/page3. Accessed Feb 2012.
4. American Cancer Society. Overview: breast cancer – what is breast cancer? 2012. http://bit.ly/Qmpa7q. Accessed Feb 2012.
5. Howe HL, Wu X, Ries LA, Cokkinides V, Ahmed F, Jemal A, et al. Annual report to the nation on the status of cancer, 1975–2003, featuring cancer among U.S. Hispanic/Latino populations. Cancer. 2006;107:1711–42.
6. National Cancer Institute. National Cancer Institute factsheet: probability of breast cancer in American women. 2010. http://www.cancer.gov/cancertopics/factsheet/detection/probability-breast-cancer. Accessed Feb 2012.
7. National Cancer Institute. What you need to know about breast cancer. 2009. http://www.cancer.gov/cancertopics/wyntk/breast/. Accessed Jan 2012.
8. American Cancer Society. Cervical cancer. 2012. http://www.cancer.org/acs/groups/cid/documents/webcontent/003094-pdf.pdf. Accessed Feb 2012.
9. National Cancer Institute. What you need to know about cervical cancer. 2008. http://www.cancer.gov/cancertopics/wyntk/cervix/. Accessed Feb 2012.
10. Texas Department of State Health Services. Texas cancer registry. Expected new cancer cases and deaths by primary site, Texas, 2012. 2011. http://www.dshs.state.tx.us/Expected-Numbers-of-Cancer-Cases-and-Deaths-Texas-2012.aspx. Accessed Feb 2012.

11. National Institues of Health. Cervical cancer fact sheet. 2010. http://report.nih.gov/NIHfactsheets/ViewFactSheet.aspx?csid=76. Accessed Feb 2012.
12. Centers for Disease Control and Prevention. HPV vaccine information for young women – fact sheet. 2011. http://www.cdc.gov/std/hpv/stdfact-hpv-vaccine-young-women.htm. Accessed May 2012.
13. Williams M, Mokry B, Risser D, Betts P, Weiss N. Cervical cancer in Texas 2006. Austin, TX: Texas Department of State Health Services; 2006.
14. National Cancer Institute. Colon and rectal cancer. 2012. http://www.cancer.gov/cancertopics/types/colon-and-rectal. Accessed Feb 2012.
15. American Cancer Society. Colorectal cancer. 2011. http://www.cancer.org/acs/groups/cid/documents/webcontent/003096-pdf.pdf. Accessed Feb 2012.
16. National Cancer Institute. What you need to know about cancer of the colon and rectum. 2006. http://www.cancer.gov/cancertopics/wyntk/colon-and-rectal. Accessed Feb 2012.
17. American Cancer Society. Colorectal cancer facts and figures 2011–2013. Atlanta: American Cancer Society; 2010.
18. American Cancer Society. Prostate cancer overview. 2012. http://www.cancer.org/acs/groups/cid/documents/webcontent/003072-pdf.pdf. Accessed Mar 2012.
19. National Cancer Institute. What you need to know about prostate cancer. 2012. http://www.cancer.gov/cancertopics/wyntk/prostate/. Accessed Mar 2012.
20. National Cancer Institute. What you need to know about lung cancer. 2012. http://www.cancer.gov/cancertopics/wyntk/lung. Accessed Mar 2012.
21. American Cancer Society. Lung cancer (non-small cell). 2012. http://www.cancer.org/acs/groups/cid/documents/webcontent/003115-pdf.pdf. Accessed Mar 2012.
22. American Cancer Society. Lung cancer (small cell). 2012. http://www.cancer.org/acs/groups/cid/documents/webcontent/003116-pdf.pdf. Accessed Mar 2012.
23. Texas Department of State Health Services. Texas cancer registry. Expected new cancer cases and deaths by primary site, Texas, 2007. 2012. http://www.dshs.state.tx.us/Expected-Numbers-of-Cancer-Cases-and-Deaths-Texas-2012.aspx. Accessed Mar 2012.
24. American Cancer Society. Liver cancer. 2011. http://www.cancer.org/acs/groups/cid/documents/webcontent/003114-pdf.pdf. Accessed Mar 2012.
25. Texas Department of State Health Services. Texas cancer registry. Expected new cancer cases and deaths by primary site, Texas, 2012. 2012. http://www.dshs.state.tx.us/Expected-Numbers-of-Cancer-Cases-and-Deaths-Texas-2012.aspx. Accessed Mar 2012.
26. National Cancer Institute. What you need to know about liver cancer. 2012. http://www.cancer.gov/cancertopics/wyntk/liver. Accessed Mar 2012.
27. American Cancer Society. Stomach cancer. 2012. http://www.cancer.org/acs/groups/cid/documents/webcontent/003141-pdf.pdf. Accessed Mar 2012.
28. National Cancer Institute. What you need to know about stomach cancer: risk factors. 2009. http://www.cancer.gov/cancertopics/wyntk/stomach. Accessed Mar 2012.
29. American Cancer Society. Gallbladder cancer. 2012. http://www.cancer.org/acs/groups/cid/documents/webcontent/003101-pdf.pdf. Accessed Mar 2012.
30. American Cancer Society. Childhood leukemia. 2010. http://www.cancer.org/acs/groups/cid/documents/webcontent/003095-pdf.pdf. Accessed Mar 2012.
31. Texas Department of State Health Services IDCU. 2009. Texas Cancer Registry Public-Use SEER*Stat Database, 1995–2009 Incidence, Texas statewide based on NPCR-CSS Submission, cut-off 11/23/11. February 2011. http://www.dshs.state.tx.us/tcr/limited-use-data.shtm. Accessed May 2013.
32. Surveillance, Epidemiology, and End Results (SEER) Program SEER*Stat Database: Incidence–SEER 13 Regs Limited-Use, Nov 2008 Sub (1992), Katrina/Rita Population Adjustment. -Linked to County Attributes -Total U.S., 1969–2009 Counties. Cancer incidence and survival among children and adolescents. National Cancer Institute, DCCPS, Surveillance Research Program, Cancer Statistics Branch, Nov 2009 Release. http://www.seer.cancer.gov. Accessed May 2013.
33. SEER Program SEER*Stat Database: Incidence–SEER 13 Regs Limited-Use, Nov 2008 Sub (1992), Katrina/Rita Population Adjustment. -Linked to County Attributes -Total U.S., 1969–2009 Counties. Cancer epidemiology in older adolescents and young adults 15 to 29 years of age including SEER incidence and survival. National Cancer Institute, DCCPS, Surveillance Research Program, Cancer Statistics Branch, Nov 2009 Release. http://www.seer.cancer.gov. Accessed May 2013.

Chapter 6
Maternal and Child Health

The health of pregnant mothers, infants, children, and adolescents is an important public health issue. Maternal and child health services such as prenatal care, primary and preventive care, immunizations, and medical treatment are vital, because they have the potential to make a difference in health status and health costs over a whole lifetime. The maternal and child health status indicators in this chapter include inadequate prenatal care, preconception health care coverage, unintended pregnancy, preconception overweight and obesity, birth defects, and infant mortality.

Inadequate Prenatal Care

Prenatal care is vitally important to the health of pregnant women and their babies. The goal of prenatal care is to identify and try to reduce risks of adverse pregnancy and birth outcomes [1]. Inadequate prenatal care has been associated with an increased risk of low birth weight births, preterm births, infant mortality, and maternal mortality [2]. Most policies and programs that attempt to improve pregnancy outcomes focus on improving the utilization of prenatal care services [3].

African-American and Hispanic mothers are more likely than non-Hispanic white mothers to obtain prenatal care late or not at all [4]. Adolescent mothers are also at a higher risk of obtaining either late or no prenatal care than mothers of other ages [2, 5]. Low income has been shown to be a major predictor of insufficient prenatal care [2].

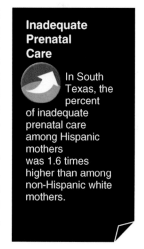

Inadequate Prenatal Care

In South Texas, the percent of inadequate prenatal care among Hispanic mothers was 1.6 times higher than among non-Hispanic white mothers.

A.G. Ramirez et al. (eds.), *The South Texas Health Status Review:*
A Health Disparities Roadmap, DOI 10.1007/978-3-319-00233-0_6, © The Author(s) 2013

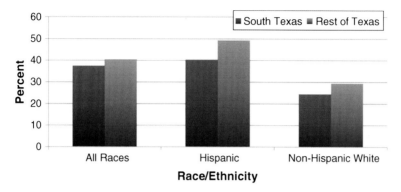

Fig. 6.1 Percent of mothers with inadequate prenatal care by location and race/ethnicity, 2005–2009. *Source*: Center for Health Statistics Data Management Team, Texas Department of State Health Services

Inadequate Prenatal Care in South Texas

In 2005–2009, an estimated 37.5 % of mothers in South Texas received inadequate prenatal care (defined as beginning prenatal care either after the first trimester of pregnancy or not receiving prenatal care at all). This estimate was slightly lower than the percent of inadequate prenatal care seen in the rest of Texas (40.4 %) (Fig. 6.1). Even though the percentage of both Hispanic and non-Hispanic white mothers receiving inadequate prenatal care in South Texas was less than their counterparts in the rest of Texas, Hispanic mothers were still at a much higher risk of having inadequate prenatal care than non-Hispanic whites (Fig. 6.1). In South Texas, the percent of inadequate prenatal care among Hispanic mothers (40.3 %) was 1.6 times higher than the percent of inadequate prenatal care among non-Hispanic white mothers (24.5 %).

In South Texas, a higher percentage of inadequate prenatal care was seen among younger maternal age groups than among the older maternal age groups. More than 50 % of the mothers in the two youngest maternal age groups (aged 10–14 and 15–17) had inadequate prenatal care, whereas only about 30 % of mothers aged 35 and older had inadequate prenatal care (Fig. 6.2).

Bexar County had a lower percentage of mothers with inadequate prenatal care (29.4 %) than all of South Texas (37.5 %). However, the Lower Rio Grande Valley area had a higher percentage of inadequate prenatal care (45.2 %) than South Texas, and the rate of inadequate prenatal care in Webb County (38.1 %) was similar to South Texas as a whole. Figure 6.3 illustrates the differences in percentages among Hispanic and non-Hispanic white mothers in each of these locations. It also shows the percent of mothers with inadequate prenatal care for African-American mothers in South Texas and Bexar County, where there were sufficient numbers to calculate an estimate for this group.

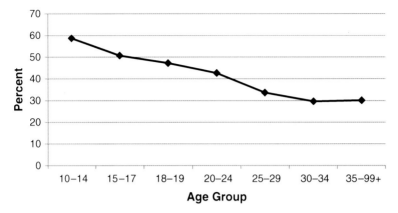

Fig. 6.2 Percent of mothers with inadequate prenatal care by age group, 2005–2009. *Source*: Center for Health Statistics Data Management Team, Texas Department of State Health Services

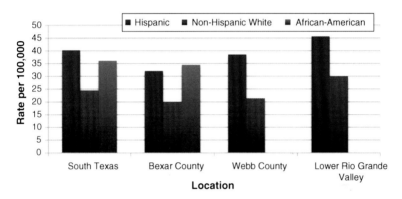

Fig. 6.3 Percent of mothers with inadequate prenatal care in selected South Texas locations by race/ethnicity, 2005–2009. *Source*: Center for Health Statistics Data Management Team, Texas Department of State Health Services

Preconception Care and Health Care Coverage Before Pregnancy

The preconception period is critically important because health conditions and behaviors during this time period can impact the health outcomes of both mother and baby. Early prenatal care (defined as prenatal care that begins during the first trimester) is also very important. However, most fetal organs have already been formed by the time of the first early prenatal care visit, and many interventions at this point are too late to prevent birth defects or other adverse maternal and infant outcomes [6, 7].

Preconception care consists of interventions that are designed to help manage, modify, and/or control risk factors that contribute to adverse maternal and infant outcomes before conception occurs. Risk factors that should be addressed in the preconception period include chronic diseases such as diabetes, high blood pressure, and heart disease; infectious diseases such as vaccine-preventable disease and HIV/AIDS; reproductive concerns such as contraception; genetic/inherited conditions such as sickle cell anemia and down syndrome; medications and medical treatment; and personal behaviors and exposures such as obesity, smoking, alcohol misuse, and folic acid supplement use [6–8].

Almost half of all pregnancies in the USA and in Texas are unintended, so preconception health care is important for all women of childbearing age and not just those planning to get pregnant. A major barrier to obtaining preconception care is lack of health care coverage, particularly for low-income women [6].

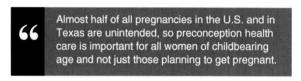

> ❝ Almost half of all pregnancies in the U.S. and in Texas are unintended, so preconception health care is important for all women of childbearing age and not just those planning to get pregnant.

Health Care Coverage in South Texas

The percent of women with no health insurance before pregnancy was statistically significantly higher in South Texas (55.5 %) than the rest of Texas (47.2 %) (Fig. 6.4).

The rates of no health insurance before pregnancy ranged from 45.2 % (among women aged 35 or older) to 58.2 % (among women aged 20–34) (Fig. 6.5).

Fig. 6.4 Estimated percent of women with no health insurance before pregnancy, by location, 2004–2009. *Source*: Texas Pregnancy Risk Assessment Monitoring System combined year dataset, 2004–2009

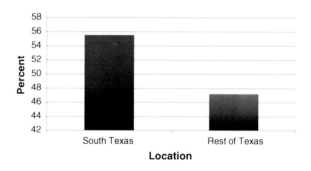

Fig. 6.5 Estimated percent of women with no health insurance before pregnancy in South Texas by age group, 2004–2009. *Source*: Texas Pregnancy Risk Assessment Monitoring System combined year dataset, 2004–2009

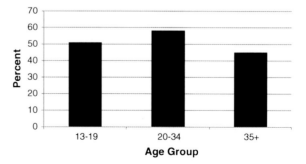

Unintended Pregnancy

An unintended pregnancy as one that is mistimed (wanted later) or unwanted at the time of conception, and an intended pregnancy is one that is wanted at the time of conception or sooner. Understanding unintended pregnancy is essential to understanding fertility, ways to prevent unwanted pregnancies, and assessing unmet needs for contraception [9, 10]. Unintended pregnancy has been associated with an increased risk of maternal morbidity and negative health behaviors during pregnancy, such as alcohol and tobacco use and delayed prenatal care, which can have adverse health effects on infants [11].

Unintended Pregnancy in South Texas

Estimates from the Texas Pregnancy Risk Assessment Monitoring System (PRAMS) indicate that the unintended pregnancy rate in 2004–2009 was the same in South Texas as in the rest of Texas (45.6 %) (Fig. 6.6).

The unintended pregnancy rate in South Texas decreased with increasing age. Women aged 13–19 had the highest rate of unintended pregnancy (66.6 %), which was twice as high as the rate among women aged 35 and older (33.3 %) (Fig. 6.7).

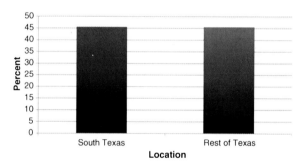

Fig. 6.6 Estimated percent of women with an unintended pregnancy, by location, 2004–2009. *Source*: Texas Pregnancy Risk Assessment Monitoring System combined year dataset, 2004–2009

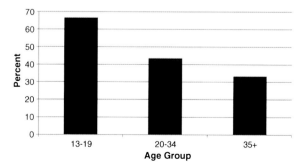

Fig. 6.7 Estimated percent of women with an unintended pregnancy in South Texas, by age group, 2004–2009. *Source*: Texas Pregnancy Risk Assessment Monitoring System combined year dataset, 2004–2009

Preconception Overweight and Obesity

The adverse health effects of obesity have been extensively studied and are well established. Obesity is associated with heart disease, stroke, breast and colon cancer, and type 2 diabetes. It is also associated with poor female reproductive health. Prepregnancy obesity is associated with numerous complications during pregnancy, such as gestational diabetes and preeclampsia [12, 13] and adverse pregnancy outcomes such as cesarean section [14, 15] and birth defects [16]. Because weight loss is not recommended during pregnancy, it is important to address weight issues during the preconception period.

Although health risks are better established among obese women, being overweight also carries risks including high blood pressure, type 2 diabetes, heart disease, and stroke. In the USA the overweight and obesity rate are rising fastest among women aged 20–34, which includes the prime childbearing ages of 20–24 [17].

Preconception Overweight and Obesity in South Texas

The prepregnancy overweight rate among women in South Texas (25.2 %) was similar to the rate among women in the rest of Texas (24.6 %). The prepregnancy obesity rate was statistically significantly higher in South Texas (25.8 %) than in the rest of Texas (20.8 %) (Fig. 6.8).

In South Texas, 23.1 % of adolescent girls aged 13–19 and approximately 25 % of women aged 20 or older were overweight before pregnancy. The prepregnancy obesity rate increased with increasing age (Fig. 6.9).

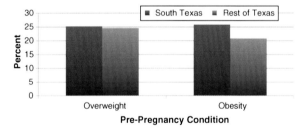

Fig. 6.8 Estimated percent of women who were overweight or obese before pregnancy, by location, 2004–2009. *Source*: Texas Pregnancy Risk Assessment Monitoring System combined year dataset, 2004–2009

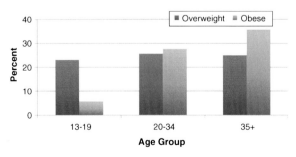

Fig. 6.9 Estimated percent of women in South Texas who were overweight or obese before pregnancy, by age group, 2004–2009. *Source*: Texas Pregnancy Risk Assessment Monitoring System combined year dataset, 2004–2009

Birth Defects

A birth defect is a problem in structure, function, or metabolism that occurs during fetal development. Birth defects can result in physical disabilities, mental disabilities, or death. In the USA, 3 % of babies are born with birth defects (about 120,000 babies annually). Birth defects are currently the leading cause of infant deaths in the USA, and babies with birth defects are at greater risk of illness and disability than babies without birth defects. Most birth defects occur during the first 3 months of pregnancy, when the baby is developing [18, 19].

Both genetic and environmental factors can play a role in the development of birth defects. Some common nongenetic risk factors include not getting enough folic acid, cigarette smoking, drinking alcohol, and maternal chronic health conditions like obesity or diabetes. However, about 70 % of all birth defects currently have unknown causes [19]. The birth defects mentioned in this section were evaluated because they are potentially preventable—studies have found associations between these birth defects and preventable factors such as low folic acid consumption, smoking, or obesity [20, 21].

Neural Tube Defects

Neural tube defects (NTDs) are a group of birth defects that have a common origin in the failure of the neural tube to develop properly during the first month of pregnancy. The three main types of NTDs are anencephaly, spina bifida, and encephalocele. Anencephaly is the most severe, involving absence of the skull and missing or reduced brain hemispheres and is always fatal. Spina bifida, the most commonly occurring NTD, is an incomplete closure of the spinal cord, and is not usually fatal. Encephalocele, the rarest NTD, is protrusion of part or all of the brain through a defect in the skull and may be fatal [22].

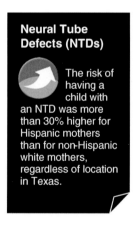

Neural Tube Defects (NTDs)

The risk of having a child with an NTD was more than 30% higher for Hispanic mothers than for non-Hispanic white mothers, regardless of location in Texas.

NTD prevalence in the USA is reported to be highest among Hispanics, followed by non-Hispanic whites, Native Americans, African-Americans, and then Asians. Studies have found that maternal periconceptional use of folic acid reduces the risk of NTDs. However, folic acid may not decrease NTD risk the same amount in all racial/ethnic groups, which suggests that genetic factors may be involved. Obesity has been associated with increased NTD prevalence, and studies also suggest that women with diabetes are at increased risk of having an infant with an NTD [22].

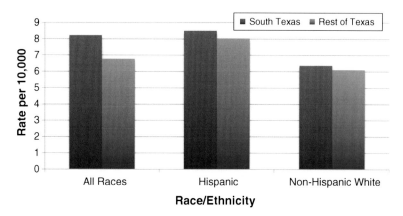

Fig. 6.10 Prevalence of neural tube defects (NTDs) by location and race/ethnicity, 2005–2009. *Source*: Texas Birth Defects Registry, 2005–2009 data

Neural Tube Defects in South Texas

The prevalence of NTDs in South Texas was 8.2 cases per 10,000 live births in 2005–2009. This was higher than the prevalence of NTDs in the rest of Texas (6.8/10,000). The risk of having a child with an NTD was more than 30 % higher for Hispanic mothers than for non-Hispanic white mothers, regardless of location in Texas (Fig. 6.10).

Oral Clefts

Oral clefts are birth defects in which the tissues of the lip or mouth do not grow together properly during fetal development. There are two types of oral clefts: cleft lip and cleft palate. Cleft lip is a groove or separation in the upper lip caused by the failure of the maxillary and median nasal processes to join together. Cleft palate is a grooved depression or opening in the roof of the mouth that occurs when the two sides of the palate do not fuse properly. Cleft lip and cleft palate can occur together, separately, or along with other defects. Cleft lip is more common than cleft palate. Oral clefts often occur together with many different chromosomal abnormalities and syndromes [23].

The latest USA estimates report that the prevalence of cleft lip with or without cleft palate is 10.6 per 10,000 live births, and the prevalence of cleft palate alone is 6.4/10,000 [24]. Oral clefts are more prevalent in male infants than female infants [23, 25]. In the USA, Asians have the highest risk of oral clefts [23, 26]. In Texas, Hispanics and non-Hispanic whites show the highest risks for cleft lip with/without cleft palate, non-Hispanic whites are highest for cleft palate, and African-Americans are lowest for both [27].

Environmental factors are considered less important than genetic factors in the etiology of oral clefts. However, *maternal smoking* has been associated with oral clefts in offspring, and studies have found that *alcohol* might increase the risk of oral clefts. Maternal intake of anticonvulsant medications and vasoactive drugs has also been associated with an increased risk of oral clefts. Maternal use of *multivitamins* has been found to reduce the risk of oral clefts, and several studies have observed a decreased risk of oral clefts with folic acid use [23].

Oral Clefts in South Texas

The prevalence of all oral clefts in South Texas (17.3/10,000) was slightly higher than the oral cleft prevalence in the rest of Texas (16.6/10,000) in 2005–2009. Race/ethnicity and sex patterns of oral cleft prevalence in South Texas were similar to what was seen in the rest of Texas.

Other Selected Birth Defects

Studies have suggested that a reduced risk of several other birth defects may be associated with multivitamin and folic acid supplement intake, including some heart defects [28, 29],limb reduction defects [30, 31], pyloric stenosis [32], and omphalocele [33]. In addition to NTDs and oral clefts, Canfield et al. (2005) observed decreases in birth prevalence for transposition of the great arteries, upper limb reduction defects, pyloric stenosis, and omphalocele after US grain fortification with folic acid. A decrease in prevalence of common truncus among Hispanics was also seen [20].

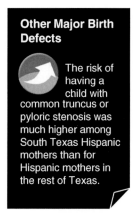

Other Major Birth Defects

The risk of having a child with common truncus or pyloric stenosis was much higher among South Texas Hispanic mothers than for Hispanic mothers in the rest of Texas.

Omphalocele is an abdominal wall defect in which an infant's bowels and other abdominal organs herniate into the umbilical cord, causing the intestines to stick out of the belly button [34, 35]. Omphalocele is associated with low birth weight, preterm birth, multiple gestation pregnancies, and intrauterine growth retardation. Mothers who are obese might be at increased risk of having an infant with omphalocele [34].

Common truncus and transposition of the great arteries are both conotruncal heart defects or outflow tract defects. With common truncus, also called truncus arteriosus, only a single blood vessel exists to carry blood both to the body and the lungs, instead of a separate aorta and pulmonary artery [36, 37]. With transposition of the great arteries, the aorta and pulmonary artery are reversed, so that the aorta carries oxygen-poor blood from the right ventricle to the rest of the body, while the pulmonary artery carries oxygen-rich blood from the left ventricle to the lungs [36, 38]. Surgery is necessary for infants with either of these birth defects to survive. *Maternal diabetes* has been associated with an increased risk of

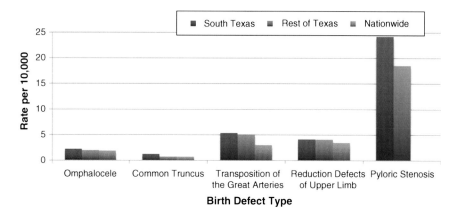

Fig. 6.11 Prevalence of selected birth defects by location. *Source*: Texas Birth Defects Registry, 2005–2009 data, 2004–2006 nationwide prevalence based on data from 11 U.S. states with active birth defects surveillance systems, obtained from Parker et al. (2010). No nationwide estimate could be found for pyloric stenosis

conotruncal defects, and *obesity* has been linked to an elevated risk of defects of the great vessels [36].

Reduction defects of the upper limb involve the congenital absence of any part of the hands or arms. The severity of these defects can vary from missing fingers to the total absence of one or both arms [27, 39]. Two general types of limb reduction defects are transverse and longitudinal defects. Transverse defects have the appearance of amputations or missing parts of the limb (e.g., a missing forearm). Longitudinal defects are missing rays of a limb (e.g., a missing radius and thumb) [27]. Limb reduction defects have been associated with maternal diabetes, exposure to pesticides, and maternal intake of a handful of medications such as thalidomide and antiseizure medicines [39].

Pyloric stenosis results from the enlargement of the pylorus muscle, which blocks the passage of food from the stomach into the small intestine. Pyloric stenosis can cause severe vomiting, weight loss, and dehydration in infants [40]. The prevalence of pyloric stenosis is highest for non-Hispanic whites and Hispanics and is lowest for African-Americans and Asians. One of the major risk factors for pyloric stenosis is a *family history* of the same defect [41].

Other Selected Birth Defects in South Texas

Figure 6.11 shows the prevalence of selected birth defects (omphalocele, common truncus, transposition of the great arteries, reduction defects of the upper limb, and pyloric stenosis) in South Texas and the rest of Texas in 2005–2009 and nationwide for the years 2004–2006. Common truncus and pyloric stenosis both had statistically significantly higher prevalence estimates in South Texas compared to the rest of Texas. The prevalence of common truncus was also significantly higher in South

Texas than the nation (Fig. 6.11) [24]. South Texas prevalence estimates for ompha-locele, transposition of the great arteries, and reduction defects of the upper limb were all similar to estimates for the rest of Texas. However, the prevalence of trans-position of the great arteries in both South Texas and the rest of Texas were signifi-cantly higher than the national prevalence. The prevalence of having a child with common truncus or pyloric stenosis was statistically significantly higher among Hispanic mothers living in South Texas than for Hispanic mothers who resided in the rest of Texas. No statistically significant differences between Hispanics and non-Hispanic whites were observed for any of these birth defects in South Texas.

Infant Mortality

Infant mortality is the death of any liveborn infant within the first year of life [4]. The infant mortality rate is an important measure of overall community health, as high infant mortality rates could be indicative of poor maternal health, inadequate access to health care, or infant malnu-trition [42]. In the USA, the infant mortality rate has greatly declined over the past few decades, from 20 infant deaths per 1,000 live births in 1970 [4] to about 6.1/1,000 in 2010 [43]. However, the USA still ranked 27th among industrialized nations in low infant mortality in 2008 [4]. This is mostly because of disparities that continue to exist

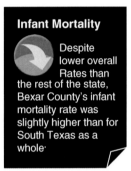

Infant Mortality

Despite lower overall Rates than the rest of the state, Bexar County's infant mortality rate was slightly higher than for South Texas as a whole·

among different race/ethnic groups in the USA [44]. The infant mortality rate in Texas has been lower than the nationwide rate since 1979. In 2008, the infant mortality rate for Texas was 6.2/1,000 compared to a national rate of 6.6/1,000 [42].

In the USA, the mortality rate for infants of African-American mothers in 2007 was 12.9/1,000, which was higher than the mortality rate for Hispanics (5.5/1,000) or non-Hispanic whites (5.6/1,000) [4]. Teenage mothers and mothers aged 40 or older have higher infant mortality rates than other maternal ages. The mortality rate is also slightly higher for male infants than for female infants [45]. The leading causes of infant mortality in the USA are birth defects, disorders related to preterm birth and low birth weight, sudden infant death syndrome, and maternal complica-tions. Risk factors for infant mortality include no prenatal care, smoking, inadequate weight gain during pregnancy, and having a repeat pregnancy within 6 months or less [45, 46].

Infant Mortality in South Texas

The infant mortality rate in South Texas from 2005 to 2009 was 5.7/1,000. The South Texas infant mortality rate was lower than in the rest of Texas (6.3/1,000).

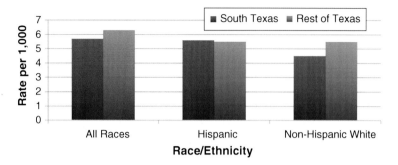

Fig. 6.12 Infant mortality rate by location and race/ethnicity, 2005–2009. *Source*: Center for Health Statistics Data Management Team, Texas Department of State Health Services

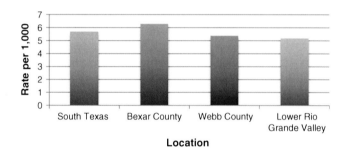

Fig. 6.13 Infant mortality rate in selected South Texas locations, 2005–2009. *Source*: Center for Health Statistics Data Management Team, Texas Department of State Health Services

The infant mortality rate for Hispanics in South Texas was similar to the rates for both Hispanics and non-Hispanic whites in the rest of Texas, and the infant mortality rate among non-Hispanic whites in South Texas was slightly lower than the mortality rate observed among non-Hispanic white infants in the rest of Texas (Fig. 6.12).

The gender pattern for infant mortality in South Texas was the same as that seen nationwide—male infants had a slightly higher mortality rate (6.0/1,000) than female infants (5.3/1,000). The infant mortality rate for Bexar County (6.3/1,000) was slightly but not statistically significantly higher than for South Texas as a whole (5.7/1,000). Webb County and the Lower Rio Grande Valley region had infant mortality rates that were slightly lower than the overall South Texas rate, but these differences were also not statistically significant (Fig. 6.13). Bexar County's infant mortality rate might have been higher because of the relatively large percent of African-Americans that reside there compared to other South Texas areas, because African-Americans have a higher infant mortality rate than Hispanics and non-Hispanic whites.

Summary: Maternal and Child Health

Table 6.1 Summary table of birth defect prevalence, percentage of inadequate prenatal care, and infant mortality rates in South Texas, the rest of Texas, and nationwide[a]

Health indicator	Prevalence, incidence, or mortality		
	South Texas	Rest of Texas	Multistate/Nation
Inadequate prenatal care	37.5 %	40.4 %	[b]
No preconception health care coverage	55.5 %	47.2 %	[b]
Unintended pregnancy	45.6 %	45.6 %	[b]
Preconception overweight	25.2 %	24.6 %	[b]
Preconception obesity	25.8 %	20.8 %	[b]
Neural tube defects	8.2 per 10,000	6.8 per 10,000	[b]
Oral clefts	17.3 per 10,000	16.6 per 10,000	[b]
Omphalocele	2.2 per 10,000	2.0 per 10,000	1.9 per 10,000
Common truncus	1.3 per 10,000	0.7 per 10,000	0.7 per 10,000
Transposition of the great arteries	5.4 per 10,000	5.1 per 10,000	3.0 per 10,000
Reduction defects of the upper limb	4.2 per 10,000	4.1 per 10,000	3.5 per 10,000
Pyloric stenosis	24.2 per 10,000	18.5 per 10,000	[b]
Infant mortality	5.7 per 1,000	6.3 per 1,000	Infant mortality

[a]Nationwide estimates were not available for all health indicators in the table
[b]Signifies that no nationwide incidence/mortality rate or prevalence of the health indicator could be found. Estimates for PRAMS health indicators (no preconception health care coverage, unintended pregnancy, preconception overweight, and preconception obesity) were calculated using 2004–2009 data, and Texas estimates for all other health indicators were calculated using 2005–2009 data. Multistate/nationwide estimates for birth defects indicators used 2004–2006 data

References

1. Liu GG. Birth outcomes and the effectiveness of prenatal care. Health Serv Res. 1998; 32:805–23.
2. Kiely JL, Kogan MD. Prenatal care. In: Wilcox LS, Marks JS, editors. From data to action: CDC's public health surveillance for women, infants, and children. Atlanta: U.S. Department of Health and Human Services, Centers for Disease Control and Prevention; 1994. p. 105–16.
3. Frick KD, Lantz PM. How well do we understand the relationship between prenatal care and birth weight? Health Serv Res. 1999;35:1063–73.
4. National Center for Health Statistics. Health, United States, 2011: with special feature on socioeconomic status and health. Hyattsville, MD: US Government Printing Office; 2012.
5. March of Dimes. Teenage pregnancy. 2009. http://bit.ly/wfBXzB. Accessed June 2012.
6. Atrash HK, Johnson K, Adams M, et al. Preconception care for improving perinatal outcomes: the time to act. Matern Child Health J. 2006;10:S3–11.
7. March of Dimes Birth Defects Foundation. March of Dimes updates: is early prenatal care too late? Contemp Ob Gyn. 2002;12:54–72.

8. Johnson K, Posner SF, Biermann J, Cordero JF, Atrash HK, Parker CS, et al. Recommendations to improve preconception health and health care – United States. MMWR Recomm Rep. 2006;55:1–23.

9. Santelli J, Rochat R, Hatfield-Timajchy K, Gilbert BC, Curtis K, Cabral R, et al. The measurement and meaning of unintended pregnancy. Perspect Sex Reprod Health. 2003;35:94–101.

10. Centers for Disease Control and Prevention. Unintended pregnancy prevention. 2012. http://www.cdc.gov/reproductivehealth/unintendedpregnancy/index.htm/. Accessed May 2012.

11. Finer L, Kost K. Unintended pregnancy rates at the state level. Perspect Sex Reprod Health. 2011;43:78–87.

12. Doherty DA, Magann EF, Francis J, Morrison JC, Newnham JP. Pre-pregnancy body mass index and pregnancy outcomes. Int J Gynecol Obstet. 2006;95:242–7.

13. Castro LC, Avina RL. Maternal obesity and pregnancy outcomes. Curr Opin Obstet Gynecol. 2002;14:601–6.

14. Crane S, Wojtowycz M, Dye T, Aubrey RH, Artal R. Association between pre-pregnancy obesity and the risk of cesarean delivery. Obstet Gynecol. 1997;89:213–6.

15. Dempsey JC, Ashiny Z, Qiu CF, Miller RS, Sorensen TK, Williams MA. Maternal pre-pregnancy overweight status and obesity as risk factors for cesarean delivery. J Matern Fetal Neonatal Med. 2005;17:179–85.

16. Centers for Disease Control and Prevention. Guidance for preventing birth defects. 2011. http://www.cdc.gov/ncbddd/birthdefects/prevention.html. Accessed May 2012.

17. Wang Y, Beydoun M. The obesity epidemic in the United States—gender, age, socioeconomic, racial/ethnic, and geographic characteristics: a systematic review and meta-regression analysis. Epidemiol Rev. 2007;29:6–28.

18. Centers for Disease Control and Prevention. Facts about birth defects. 2011. http://www.cdc.gov/ncbddd/birthdefects/facts.html. Accessed Apr 2012.

19. March of Dimes. Quick reference: birth defects. 2010. http://www.milesforbabies.org/professionals/14332_1206.asp. Accessed Apr 2012.

20. Canfield MA, Collins JS, Botto LD, Williams LJ, Mai CT, Kirby RS, et al. Changes in the birth prevalence of selected birth defects after grain fortification with folic acid in the United States: findings from a multi-state population-based study. Birth Defects Res A Clin Mol Teratol. 2005;73:679–89.

21. Texas Department of State Health Services. Birth defects risk factor series. 2011. http://www.dshs.state.tx.us/birthdefects/bd_risk_main.shtm. Accessed Apr 2012.

22. Texas Department of State Health Services. Birth defects risk factor series: neural tube defects. 2006. http://www.dshs.state.tx.us/birthdefects/risk/risk7-NTDS.shtm. Accessed Apr 2012.

23. Texas Department of State Health Services. Birth defects risk factor series: oral clefts. 2005. http://www.dshs.state.tx.us/birthdefects/risk/risk-oralclefts.shtm. Accessed Apr 2012.

24. Parker SE, Mai CT, Canfield MA, Rickard R, Wang Y, Meyer RE, et al. Updated national birth prevalence estimates for selected birth defects in the United States, 2004-2006. Birth Defects Res A Clin Mol Teratol. 2010;88:1008–16.

25. Dental, Oral and Craniofacial Data Resource Center. Oral Health U.S., 2002. Bethesda, MD: Dental, Oral and Craniofacial Data Resource Center; 2007.

26. March of Dimes. Quick reference: cleft lip and cleft palate. 2007. http://www.milesforbabies.org/professionals/14332_1210.asp. Accessed Apr 2012.

27. Birth Defects Epidemiology and Surveillance Branch. Report of birth defects among 2000–2009 deliveries. Publication No. 58-13601. Texas Department of State Health Services; 2012.

28. Botto L, Khoury M, Mulinare J, Erickson J. Periconceptional multivitamin use and the occurrence of conotruncal heart defects: results from a population-based, case-control study. Pediatrics. 1996;98:911–7.

29. Shaw G, O'Malley C, Wasserman C, Tolarova M, Lammer E. Maternal periconceptional use of multivitamins and reduced risk for conotruncal heart defects and limb deficiencies among offspring. Am J Med Genet. 1995;59:536–45.

30. Werler M, Hayes C, Louik C, Shapiro S, Mitchell A. Multivitamin supplementation and risk of birth defects. Am J Epidemiol. 1999;150:675–82.

31. Yang Q, Khoury M, Erickson J, James L, Waters G, Berry R. Does periconceptional multivitamin use reduce the risk for limb deficiency in offspring? Epidemiology. 1997;8:157–61.

32. Czeizel A. Periconceptional folic acid containing multivitamin supplementation. Eur J Obstet Gynecol Reprod Biol. 1998;78:151–61.

33. Botto L, Mulinare J, Erickson J. Occurrence of omphalocele in relation to maternal multivitamin use: a population-based study. Pediatrics. 2002;109:904–8.

34. Texas Department of State Health Services. Birth defects risk factor series: omphalocele. 2009. http://www.dshs.state.tx.us/birthdefects/risk/risk8-omphalocele.shtm. Accessed Apr 2012.

35. Medline Plus. Omphalocele. 2011. http://www.nlm.nih.gov/medlineplus/ency/article/000994.htm. Accessed Apr 2012.

36. Texas Department of State Health Services. Birth defects risk factor series: conotruncal heart defects. 2007. http://www.dshs.state.tx.us/birthdefects/risk/risk15-conotrncl.shtm. Accessed May 2012.

37. American Heart Association. Truncus arteriosus. 2012. http://www.heart.org/HEARTORG/Conditions/CongenitalHeartDefects/AboutCongenitalHeartDefects/Truncus-Arteriosus_UCM_307040_Article.jsp#.T4Xv9tmrZ8E. Accessed Apr 2012.

38. Mayo Clinic Staff. Transposition of the great arteries. Mayo Clinic. 2010. http://www.mayoclinic.com/health/transposition-of-the-great-arteries/DS00733. Accessed Apr 2012.

39. Mekdeci B, Schettler T. Birth defects and the environment. The collaborative on health and the environment. 2004. http://www.healthandenvironment.org/birth_defects/peer_reviewed. Accessed Apr 2012.

40. Mayo Clinic Staff. Pyloric stenosis: introduction. Mayo Clinic. 2010. http://www.mayoclinic.com/health/pyloric-stenosis/DS00815. Accessed Apr 2012.

41. Texas Department of State Health Services. Birth defects risk factor series: pyloric stenosis. 2002. http://www.dshs.state.tx.us/birthdefects/risk/risk21-pyl_sten.shtm. Accessed Apr 2012.

42. Texas Department of State Health Services. Texas infant mortality rates. 2012. http://soupfin.tdh.state.tx.us/imr.htm. Accessed May 2012.

43. Murphy SL, Xu J, Kochanek KD. Deaths: preliminary data for 2010. Natl Vital Stat Rep 2012;60.

44. MacDorman MF, Mathews TJ. Understanding racial and ethnic disparities in U.S. infant mortality rates. NCHS Data Brief 2011;74.

45. Mathews T, MacDorman MF. Infant mortality statistics from the 2004 period linked birth/infant death data set. Natl Vital Stat Rep 2007;55

46. U S Department of Health and Human Services. Fact sheet: preventing infant mortality. 2006. http://www.hhs.gov/news/factsheet/infant.html. Accessed May 2012.

Chapter 7
Chronic Diseases

Chronic diseases, such as diabetes, heart disease, stroke, and cancer, are currently the leading causes of both death and disability in the USA. It is estimated that 70 % of all deaths nationwide are due to chronic illnesses (1.7 million deaths each year), and 133 million Americans were living with a chronic disease in 2005. Although chronic diseases are some of the most prevalent and costly health problems in the USA, they are also largely preventable. Healthy behaviors, such as getting enough exercise, eating right, and avoiding tobacco, can help to prevent many chronic diseases [1]. In this chapter, chronic disease mortality rates are presented as age-adjusted rates; prevalence of chronic diseases are presented as crude estimates.

Diabetes

Diabetes is a group of diseases that result from the body's inability to produce or correctly use insulin, a hormone that regulates sugar metabolism [2, 3]. Type 2 diabetes is the most common form of diabetes, accounting for 90–95 % of all diagnosed cases. Type 2 diabetes usually results from insulin resistance, a disorder in which the body does not properly use insulin, as well as problems with insulin production [3]. Diabetes is associated with numerous serious health complications such as cardiovascular disease, blindness, kidney failure, nervous system damage, and amputations [2, 3]. African-Americans, Hispanics, Native Americans, and Asian Americans are at higher risk for Type 2 diabetes than are non-Hispanic whites [2]. Risk factors for Type 2 diabetes include overweight and obesity, physical inactivity, a history of gestational diabetes, and a family history of diabetes [2, 3].

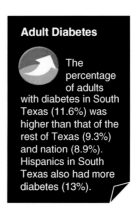

Adult Diabetes

The percentage of adults with diabetes in South Texas (11.6%) was higher than that of the rest of Texas (9.3%) and nation (8.9%). Hispanics in South Texas also had more diabetes (13%).

A.G. Ramirez et al. (eds.), *The South Texas Health Status Review:*
A Health Disparities Roadmap, DOI 10.1007/978-3-319-00233-0_7, © The Author(s) 2013

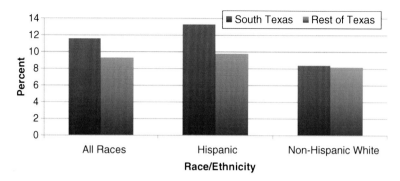

Fig. 7.1 Estimated percent of the adult population with diabetes by location and race/ethnicity, 2007–2010. *Source*: Texas Behavioral Risk Factor Surveillance System Combined Year Dataset, Statewide BRFSS Survey, 2007–2010

Diabetes Prevalence

An estimated 8.3 % (or 25.8 million people) of the US population had diabetes in 2010. If trends continue, an estimated one in three US adults will have diabetes by 2050 [2]. In Texas, approximately 1.7 million adults (aged 18 or older) were living with diagnosed diabetes in 2009 [4]. Type 2 diabetes, which accounts for the large majority of diabetes cases, is usually associated with older age [2]. Approximately 1.9 million new cases of diabetes were diagnosed in people aged 20 or older in 2010 [2].

Diabetes Prevalence in South Texas

An estimated 11.6 % of adults who live in South Texas have been diagnosed with diabetes. The percent of adults with diabetes in South Texas was higher than the estimated percent with diabetes in the rest of Texas (9.3 %) and national BRFSS 2007–2010 estimates (8.9 %). Hispanics in South Texas had a higher prevalence of diabetes than did Hispanics in the rest of Texas. Hispanics also had a significantly higher prevalence of diabetes than non-Hispanic whites in South Texas (Fig. 7.1).

Age patterns for diabetes prevalence in South Texas were the same as seen nationwide; the prevalence of diabetes in South Texas increased with age. For those aged 30 or older, the prevalence of diabetes was statistically significantly higher among Hispanics than among non-Hispanic whites. An estimated 34 % of Hispanic adults aged 65 and older in South Texas were diagnosed with diabetes in 2007–2010 (Fig. 7.2).

Overall, the prevalence of diabetes was similar among South Texas metropolitan and nonmetropolitan counties (11.4 % and 12.4 %, respectively).

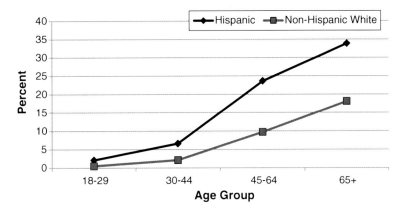

Fig. 7.2 Estimated percent of the adult South Texas population with diabetes by age group and race/ethnicity, 2007–2010. *Source*: Texas Behavioral Risk Factor Surveillance System Combined Year Dataset, Statewide BRFSS Survey, 2007–2010

Diabetes Mortality

Nationally, diabetes was the seventh leading cause of death in 2007 [2] and the sixth leading cause of death from 2002 to 2007 in Texas [4]. This ranking was based on death certificates that listed diabetes as the underlying cause of death. Mortality from diabetes is believed to be underreported; it is listed as a contributing factor more often than it is listed as an underlying factor, and diabetes is often not listed at all on the death certificate. In 2007, including diabetes as an underlying cause of death and a contributing factor, there were 231,404 deaths due to diabetes in the USA [5].

Diabetes Mortality in South Texas

The 2005–2009 age-adjusted diabetes mortality rate in South Texas (with diabetes reported either as an underlying or contributing cause of death) was 170.9 deaths per 100,000 persons. This rate was significantly higher than the age-adjusted diabetes mortality rate in the rest of Texas (82.1/100,000). Hispanics had a higher diabetes mortality rate than non-Hispanic whites, both in South Texas and the rest of Texas. The age-adjusted diabetes mortality rate for Hispanics in South Texas (219.6/100,000) was twice as high as the rate for Hispanics in the rest of Texas (108.92/100,000), and non-Hispanic whites in South Texas also had a higher age-adjusted diabetes mortality rate than did non-Hispanic whites in the rest of Texas (Fig. 7.3).

As with diabetes prevalence, the diabetes mortality rate in South Texas increased with age, and diabetes mortality rates were higher for Hispanics than for non-Hispanic whites among those aged 35 and older. South Texas Hispanics aged 75 or older had a diabetes mortality rate of 1,981.5/100,000 (Fig. 7.4).

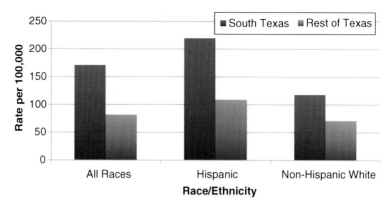

Fig. 7.3 Age-adjusted mortality rates for diabetes as an underlying or contributing cause, by location and race/ethnicity, 2005–2009. *Source*: Center for Health Statistics Data Management Team, Texas Department of State Health Services

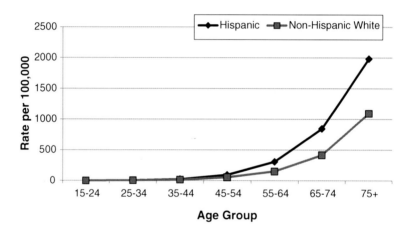

Fig. 7.4 South Texas age-adjusted mortality rates for diabetes as an underlying or contributing cause, by age group and race/ethnicity, 2005–2009. *Source*: Center for Health Statistics Data Management Team, Texas Department of State Health Services

In South Texas, males had a higher diabetes mortality rate (189.4/100,000) than females (155.6/100,000). Residents of South Texas metropolitan counties had a higher diabetes mortality rate (173.1/100,000) than did residents of nonmetropolitan counties (159.2/100,000).

Bexar County and Webb County both had higher diabetes mortality rates than South Texas, whereas the Lower Rio Grande Valley region had a lower mortality rate than South Texas (Fig. 7.5).

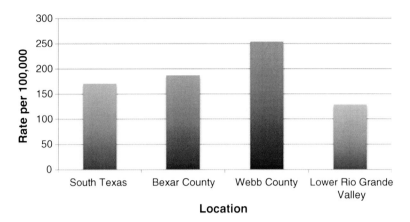

Fig. 7.5 Age-adjusted mortality rates for diabetes as an underlying or contributing cause in selected South Texas locations, 2005–2009. *Source*: Center for Health Statistics Data Management Team, Texas Department of State Health Services

Cardiovascular Disease

Cardiovascular disease (CVD) is a general term given to any disease affecting the heart or blood vessels. CVD is the leading cause of death in the USA [6]. The American Heart Association estimated that 82.6 million Americans (more than one in three) were living with one or more forms of CVD in 2008. About 32.8 % of all deaths in the USA (811,940) were attributable to CVD in 2008 [7]. Heart disease and cerebrovascular disease (stroke) are the two main causes of CVD death [6].

Heart Disease Mortality

Heart disease is the leading cause of death in the USA, accounting for 25 % of all US deaths in 2008 [6]. It is the leading cause of death for both US men and women, as well as the leading cause of death for African-Americans, Hispanics, and Whites [8]. In the USA in 2007–2009, African-American adults had the highest age-adjusted heart disease death rate (239.9/100,000), followed by whites (182.9/100,000) and Hispanics (128.6/100,000) [9]. Coronary heart disease, which can lead to heart attacks, is the most common form of heart disease in the USA; however, several other heart conditions also fall under the term heart disease [8].

The risk of heart disease, and subsequently heart disease mortality, increases with age. Approximately 82 % of coronary heart disease deaths occur among those aged 65 or older. Men have a greater risk of heart disease than women, especially at younger ages [10]. Major risk factors for heart disease include high blood pressure, high blood cholesterol levels, cigarette smoking, and diabetes [8, 10]. About 65 %

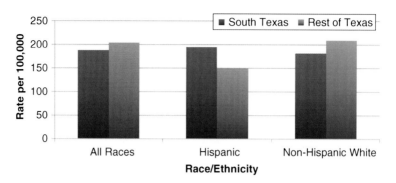

Fig. 7.6 Heart disease mortality rates in South Texas and the rest of Texas by race/ethnicity, 2005–2009. *Source*: Center for Health Statistics Data Management Team, Texas Department of State Health Services

of diabetics die of some form of heart or blood vessel disease [10, 11]. In addition, poor diet and physical inactivity have been linked to heart disease, probably because they are related to the major risk factors listed above. Similarly, obesity is an indirect risk factor for heart disease, because it is linked to high cholesterol, high blood pressure, and diabetes [8, 10].

Heart Disease Mortality in South Texas

Overall, South Texas had a lower age-adjusted heart disease mortality rate (187.9/100,000) than did the rest of Texas (204.1/100,000). Although non-Hispanic whites in South Texas had a lower heart disease mortality rate than non-Hispanic whites in the rest of Texas, the opposite was seen for Hispanics (Fig. 7.6). South Texas Hispanics had a higher mortality rate than Hispanics in the rest of Texas. Unlike in the rest of Texas and nation, where Hispanics die less frequently from heart disease than non-Hispanic whites, Hispanics in South Texas had a slightly higher heart disease mortality rate than their non-Hispanic white counterparts (Fig. 7.6).

Gender and age patterns for heart disease mortality in South Texas were the same as seen nationwide. For all races combined, nonmetropolitan counties in South Texas had a higher age-adjusted heart disease mortality rate than did metropolitan counties (Fig. 7.7). Hispanics in nonmetropolitan counties also had a higher heart disease mortality rate (220.5/100,000) than did Hispanics in metropolitan counties (190.2/100,000), and this difference in rates was larger than for all races combined. On the other hand, the mortality rate among non-Hispanic whites was only slightly and not statistically significantly higher in nonmetropolitan counties than in metropolitan counties (Fig. 7.7).

The average annual age-adjusted heart disease mortality rates for Bexar County (183.0/100,000) and the Lower Rio Grande Valley area (182.9/100,000) were both similar to the mortality rate for South Texas as a whole (187.9/100,000). However, Webb County's heart disease mortality rate (209.4/100,000) was higher than the overall South Texas rate (Fig. 7.8).

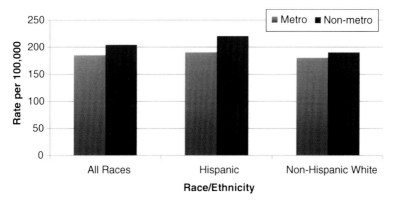

Fig. 7.7 Heart disease mortality rates in South Texas, by county designation and race/ethnicity, 2005–2009. *Source*: Center for Health Statistics Data Management Team, Department of State Health Services

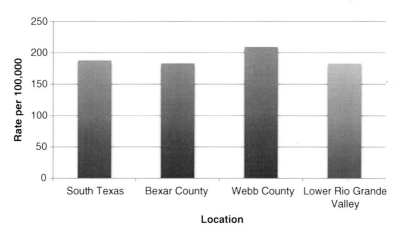

Fig. 7.8 Heart disease mortality rates in selected South Texas locations, 2005–2009. *Source*: Center for Health Statistics Data Management Team, Texas Department of State Health Services

Cerebrovascular Disease Mortality

Cerebrovascular disease, more commonly known as stroke, is the fourth leading cause of death in the USA [6, 12]. A stroke is characterized by neurological damage that occurs either when the brain's blood supply is blocked or when a blood vessel in the brain bursts [13]. About 610,000 new strokes occur each year in the USA [7, 13], causing the death of more than 128,000 people [12] and also causing long-term disability in others. Individuals who have had strokes can sustain major disabilities such as paralysis or speech problems [14]. Approximately 75 % of all strokes occur among individuals aged 65 or older [13]. Men have a slightly higher

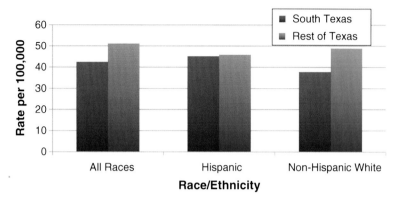

Fig. 7.9 Stroke mortality rates in South Texas and the rest of Texas by race/ethnicity, 2005–2009. *Source*: Center for Health Statistics Data Management Team, Texas Department of State Health Services

age-adjusted prevalence and incidence of stroke than women, but women have a greater lifetime risk of stroke [7, 15].

Major risk factors for stroke include high blood pressure, heart disease, diabetes, and cigarette smoking [7, 13]. Smoking doubles the risk of cerebrovascular disease, and the risk of stroke for individuals with diabetes is at least doubled compared to those without diabetes. Other risk factors for stroke include pregnancy and physical inactivity [7].

Cerebrovascular Disease Mortality in South Texas

Overall, South Texas had a lower annual age-adjusted cerebrovascular disease mortality rate (42.5/100,000) than did the rest of Texas (51.1/100,000) from 2005 to 2009. The non-Hispanic white population in South Texas also had a lower mortality rate than non-Hispanic whites in the rest of Texas. No difference in rates was seen in the Hispanic population by location (South Texas vs. the rest of Texas). Hispanics had a higher stroke mortality rate than non-Hispanic whites in South Texas (Fig. 7.9).

The cerebrovascular mortality age trend in South Texas was similar to the age trend observed nationally. Overall, stroke mortality rates in South Texas were higher for males than for females. Among Hispanics, males also had a higher stroke mortality rate than females, and this difference in mortality rates was larger than for all races combined. Among non-Hispanic whites, however, females had a very slightly but not significantly higher stroke mortality rate than males (Fig. 7.10).

Webb County and Bexar County had higher mortality rates (49.1/100,000 and 45.5/100,000 respectively) than South Texas as a whole (42.5/100,000), and the Lower Rio Grande Valley region had a lower mortality rate (33.4/100,000) than all of South Texas.

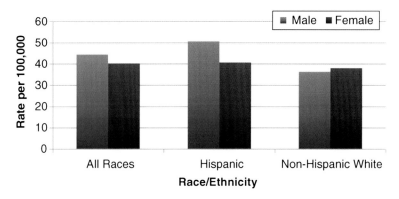

Fig. 7.10 Stroke mortality rates in South Texas by sex and race/ethnicity, 2005–2009. *Source:* Center for Health Statistics Data Management Team, Texas Department of State Health Services

Asthma

Asthma is a chronic disease of the respiratory system that is characterized by episodes of airway inflammation, usually in response to one or more triggers. If not properly managed, asthma can be life threatening. The prevalence of asthma in the USA appears to have increased slightly over the past few years. An estimated 24.6 million Americans, of which 7.1 million were children, had asthma in 2009 [16]. Asthma is one of the most common chronic diseases among children and is the third leading cause of hospitalization in children younger than 15 years of age [17].

Among all US age groups, the highest prevalence of asthma in 2009 occurred in people aged 5–17 (almost 11 %). Among adults, asthma prevalence is higher in women than in men. This trend is reversed for children and adolescents, however; among those younger than 18, boys have a higher prevalence of asthma than girls. In 2009, prevalence of current asthma in the USA was highest in African-Americans (11.2 %), followed by non-Hispanic whites (8.2 %) and Hispanics (6.3 %) [16].

Current Asthma in South Texas Adults

An estimated 6.4 % of adult South Texas residents had asthma in 2007–2010. This percentage was slightly lower than the estimate of current asthma in the rest of Texas (7.6 %). Current asthma rates in South Texas and the rest of Texas were lower than the current asthma estimate nationwide (8.4 %). In South Texas, a greater percentage of non-Hispanic whites (7.5 %) were estimated to currently have asthma than Hispanics (5.7 %), although this difference was not statistically significant. The prevalence of current asthma was almost twice as high in females (8.4 %) than males (4.4 %).

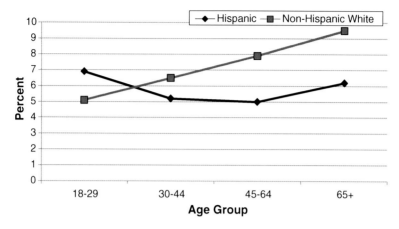

Fig. 7.11 Estimated prevalence of current asthma among South Texas adults by age group and race/ethnicity, 2007–2010. *Source*: Texas Behavioral Risk Factor Surveillance System Combined Year Dataset, Statewide BRFSS Survey, 2007–2010

The current asthma prevalence age trends for Hispanic and non-Hispanic white adults were somewhat different from each other. Among non-Hispanic whites, current asthma prevalence estimates increased with age, whereas this trend was not seen among Hispanics. Although non-Hispanic whites had higher current asthma prevalence estimates than Hispanics among those aged 30 and older, this difference was only statistically significant for those aged 45–64 (Fig. 7.11).

Summary

Table 7.1 Summary table of crude prevalence or age-adjusted mortality rates in South Texas, the rest of Texas, and nationwide[a] for each of the chronic disease indicators analyzed

Health indicator	Prevalence or mortality rate		
	South Texas	Rest of Texas	Nationwide
Diabetes prevalence, 2007–2010	11.6 %	9.3 %	8.9 %
Diabetes mortality, 2005–2009	170.9/100,000	82.1/100,000	[b]
Heart disease mortality, 2005–2009	187.9/100,000	204.1/100,000	[b]
Cerebrovascular disease mortality, 2005–2009	42.5/100,000	51.1/100,000	[b]
Asthma prevalence, 2007–2010	6.4 %	7.6 %	8.4 %

[a]Nationwide estimates were not available for all health indicators in the table
[b]Signifies that no nationwide mortality rate could be found for the health indicator

References

1. Centers for Disease Control and Prevention. Chronic disease prevention . 2012. http://www.cdc.gov/nccdphp/. Accessed May 2012.
2. Centers for Disease Control and Prevention. Diabetes at a glance. 2011. Centers for Disease Control and Prevention. http://www.cdc.gov/chronicdisease/resources/publications/aag/pdf/2011/Diabetes-AAG-2011-508.pdf. Accessed May 2012.
3. American Diabetes Association. Diabetes basics. 2012. http://www.diabetes.org/diabetes-basics/. Accessed May 2012.
4. Texas Diabetes Council. Diabetes and disparity: a plan to prevent and control diabetes in Texas, 2012–2013. Publication No. 45-10524. Austin: Texas Department of State Health Services; 2011.
5. Centers for Disease Control and Prevention. National diabetes fact sheet: national estimates and general information on diabetes in the United States, 2011. Atlanta: U.S. Department of Health and Human Services, Centers for Disease Control and Prevention; 2011.
6. Miniño AM, Murphy SL, Xu J, Kochanek KD. Deaths: final data for 2008. Natl Vital Stat Rep. 2011;59:1–126.
7. Roger VL, Go AS, Loyd-Jones DM, Benjamin EJ, Berry JD, Borden WB, et al. Heart disease and stroke statistics – 2012 update: a report from the American Heart Association. Circulation. 2012;125:e2–220.
8. Centers for Disease Control and Prevention. Heart disease. 2012. http://www.cdc.gov/HeartDisease/. Accessed May 2012.
9. Centers for Disease Control and Prevention. Health data interactive: 2007–2009. http://205.207.175.93/HDI/ReportFolders/reportFolders.aspx. Accessed May 2012.
10. American Heart Association. Understand your risk of heart attack. 2012. http://www.heart.org/HEARTORG/Conditions/HeartAttack/UnderstandYourRiskofHeartAttack/Understand-Your-Risk-of-Heart-Attack_UCM_002040_Article.jsp. Accessed May 2012.
11. American Heart Association. Cardiovascular disease and diabetes. 2012. http://www.heart.org/HEARTORG/Conditions/Diabetes/WhyDiabetesMatters/Cardiovascular-Disease-Diabetes_UCM_313865_Article.jsp. Accessed May 2012.
12. Centers for Disease Control and Prevention. Leading causes of death. 2012. http://www.cdc.gov/nchs/fastats/lcod.htm. Accessed May 2012.
13. Centers for Disease Control and Prevention. Stroke. 2012. http://www.cdc.gov/Stroke/. Accessed May 2012.
14. National Institute of Neurological Disorders and Stroke. Post-stroke rehabilitation fact sheet. 2011. http://www.ninds.nih.gov/disorders/stroke/poststrokerehab.htm. Accessed May 2012.
15. Fang J, Shaw KM, George MG. Prevalence of stroke – United States, 2006–2010. MMWR Morb Mortal Wkly Rep. 2012;61:379–82.
16. American Lung Association. Trends in asthma morbidity and mortality. 2011. http://www.lung.org/finding-cures/our-research/trend-reports/asthma-trend-report.pdf. Accessed May 2012.
17. American Lung Association. Asthma & children fact sheet. 2011. http://www.lung.org/lung-disease/asthma/resources/facts-and-figures/asthma-children-fact-sheet.html. Accessed May 2012.

Chapter 8
Behavioral Risk Factors in Adults

Behavioral risk factors are behaviors that increase the possibility of disease, such as smoking, alcohol use, bad eating habits, and not getting enough exercise. Because they are behaviors, it is possible for individuals to modify these risk factors to help prevent many types of chronic diseases and premature death.

Obesity

The rising prevalence of overweight and obesity among both adults and children are of serious concern nationwide. More than one-third of US adults are obese [1]. Nationwide, the prevalence of obesity among children and adolescents has tripled compared to the prevalence observed just one generation ago [2]. In Texas, 31 % of adults are estimated to be obese. Texas is one of only 12 US states with a percentage of obese adults exceeding 30 % [3]. Approximately one-third of children in Texas are either overweight or obese [4, 5]. This is alarming, because overweight and obese children have an increased risk of obesity in adulthood [6, 7].

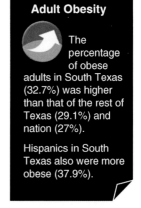

Adult Obesity

The percentage of obese adults in South Texas (32.7%) was higher than that of the rest of Texas (29.1%) and nation (27%).

Hispanics in South Texas also were more obese (37.9%).

The amount of body fat in an individual is usually estimated by calculating their body mass index (BMI), which takes both weight and height into account. Adults with a BMI of 30 or greater are considered obese [1]. Obesity is associated with increased risk of a host of health problems, including heart disease, stroke, hypertension, hypercholesterolemia, diabetes, osteoarthritis, and several different types of cancer [8, 9]. Because overweight and obesity are usually caused by an energy imbalance (consuming more calories than are used) over a long period of time, poor eating habits and not getting enough physical exercise are two major contributing factors for these conditions [9].

A.G. Ramirez et al. (eds.), *The South Texas Health Status Review:*
A Health Disparities Roadmap, DOI 10.1007/978-3-319-00233-0_8, © The Author(s) 2013

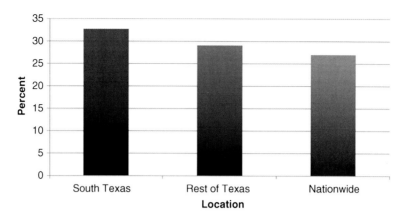

Fig. 8.1 Estimated percent of the adult (18+) population with obesity by location, 2007–2010. *Source*: Texas Behavioral Risk Factor Surveillance System Combined Year Dataset, Statewide BRFSS Survey, 2007–2010, CDC Behavioral Risk Factor Surveillance System, Nationwide BRFSS Survey, 2007–2010

African-American and Mexican-American adults in the USA have higher obesity rates than non-Hispanic white adults [3]. Prevalence of obesity in the USA generally increases with age; adolescents have a higher prevalence of obesity than do children, and older adults tend to have a higher prevalence of obesity than younger adults. In 2009–2010, there was no significant difference in the nationwide prevalence of obesity between women and men [1].

Obesity in South Texas

In 2007–2010, 32.7 % of adults who lived in South Texas were obese. The prevalence of obesity in South Texas was higher than the prevalence of obesity in the rest of Texas (29.1 %) or nation (27.0 %) (Fig. 8.1).

In South Texas, a higher prevalence of obesity was seen in Hispanic adults (37.9 %) than in non-Hispanic whites (24.6 %). Hispanics in South Texas also had a higher obesity prevalence (37.9 %) than Hispanics in the rest of Texas (34.2 %) (Fig. 8.2).

Age and gender obesity prevalence patterns in South Texas were similar to national trends. The highest age-specific obesity prevalence was observed among adults aged 30–64 (about 36 %). For non-Hispanic whites, the prevalence of obesity was very similar in South Texas metropolitan and nonmetropolitan counties. However, the percent of Hispanics who were obese in nonmetropolitan counties was higher than the percent of obese Hispanics in metropolitan counties (Fig. 8.3).

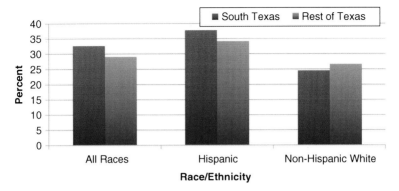

Fig. 8.2 Estimated percent of the adult population with obesity in South Texas and the rest of Texas by race/ethnicity, 2007–2010. *Source*: Texas Behavioral Risk Factor Surveillance System Combined Year Dataset, Statewide BRFSS Survey, 2007–2010

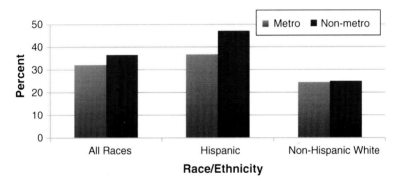

Fig. 8.3 Estimated percent of the adult population with obesity in South Texas by county designation and race/ethnicity, 2007–2010. *Source*: Texas Behavioral Risk Factor Surveillance System Combined Year Dataset, Statewide BRFSS Survey, 2007–2010

Physical Activity

Engaging in regular physical activity can help reduce the risk of conditions such as obesity, heart disease, diabetes, hypertension, colon cancer, and premature mortality [10]. Regular, moderate levels of exercise each day can lead to improved health and well-being. The CDC recommends that adults either engage in moderate-intensity physical activity for at least 150 min (2 h and 30 min) per week, or engage in vigorous-intensity physical activity for at least 75 min (1 h and 15 min) 3 or more days per week [10, 11].

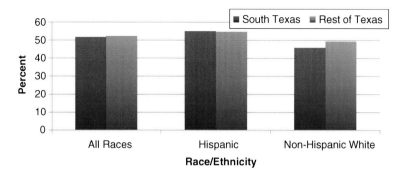

Fig. 8.4 Estimated prevalence of inadequate physical activity among adults (18+) by location and race/ethnicity, 2007 and 2009. *Source*: Texas Behavioral Risk Factor Surveillance System Combined Year Dataset, Statewide BRFSS Survey, 2007 and 2009

Even though the benefits of physical activity are well known, more than 50 % of all adults in the USA get less than the recommended amount of physical activity, and 25 % are not active at all during their leisure time. Nationally, fewer women than men get sufficient physical activity. Activity also decreases with age; older individuals are less likely to get adequate physical activity. Inadequate physical activity is more common among adults with lower incomes and less education. Inadequate physical activity is not only a problem for adults—an estimated two-thirds of high-school-aged youth are not engaged in recommended physical activity levels [12].

Inadequate Physical Activity in South Texas

An estimated 51.8 % of adults in South Texas got inadequate physical activity (did not meet weekly recommendations for moderate or vigorous physical activity) during 2007 and 2009. This percentage was similar to the estimated prevalence of inadequate physical activity in the rest of Texas (Fig. 8.4). Adults in South Texas also had a prevalence of inadequate physical activity similar to the national 2007 and 2009 BRFSS estimate (51.1 %).

Hispanics in South Texas had a prevalence of inadequate physical activity (55.1 %) that was similar to Hispanics in the rest of Texas (54.8 %). In both South Texas and the rest of Texas, the percent of Hispanics who did not engage in sufficient physical activity was higher than the percent for non-Hispanic whites (Fig. 8.4).

Inadequate physical activity gender and age patterns among South Texas adults were similar to those reported nationwide. In South Texas, inadequate physical activity generally increased with age among both Hispanic and non-Hispanic white adults. Hispanics aged 30–44 and 45–64 had higher prevalences of inadequate physical activity than did non-Hispanic whites of the same age groups (Fig. 8.5).

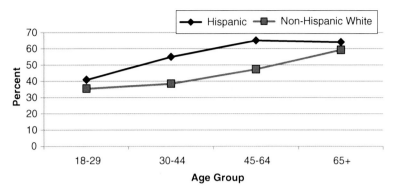

Fig. 8.5 Estimated prevalence of inadequate physical activity among South Texas adults by age group and race/ethnicity, 2007 and 2009. *Source*: Texas Behavioral Risk Factor Surveillance System Combined Year Dataset, Statewide BRFSS Survey, 2007 and 2009

Nutrition

Good nutrition can help to lower the risk of chronic diseases such as stroke, heart disease, some cancers, osteoporosis, and diabetes [12]. Adequate fruit and vegetable consumption is a key component of good nutrition. Fruits and vegetables contain vitamins, minerals, and fiber that are critical to good health. It is likely that people who consume more generous amounts of fruits and vegetables have a reduced risk of cardiovascular disease and certain cancers than people who eat only small amounts of fruits and vegetables [13]. The U.S. Department of Health and Human Services and the U.S. Department of Agriculture recommend that adults with a 2,000-calorie intake eat 2 cups of fruit and 2½ cups of vegetables every day [14].

Less than one-fourth of adults in the USA had adequate fruit and vegetable consumption (ate five or more servings of fruits and vegetables each day) in 2009. Nationwide, a higher percentage of women had adequate fruit and vegetable consumption than men. Inadequate fruit and vegetable consumption was higher for African-American and Hispanic adults than for other racial/ethnic groups. Younger adult age groups (aged 18–44) were more likely to consume inadequate amounts of fruits and vegetables than older adults (ages 45 and older) [15].

Inadequate Fruit and Vegetable Consumption in South Texas

An estimated 76.2 % of adults in South Texas had inadequate fruit and vegetable consumption (ate less than five servings of fruits and vegetables per day) during 2007 and 2009. This percentage was similar to the percent of adults with inadequate fruit and vegetable consumption in the rest of Texas (75.1 %) and nationwide (75.8 %).

Sex, age, and race/ethnicity patterns of inadequate fruit and vegetable consumption in South Texas were similar to those seen nationwide. Hispanic adults had a higher prevalence of inadequate fruit and vegetable consumption (79.5 %) than non-Hispanic whites (73.4 %), adults in older age groups had a lower prevalence of inadequate fruit and vegetable consumption, and men had a higher percentage of inadequate fruit and vegetable consumption (79.9 %) than women (72.7 %).

Cigarette Smoking Behaviors

Smoking cigarettes harms nearly every organ in the body and can cause many adverse health effects including cancer, cardiovascular disease, and respiratory diseases [16]. Cigarette smoking is currently the leading preventable cause of death in the USA. During 2000–2004, cigarette smoking and exposure to tobacco smoke resulted in 1 out of every 5 deaths (443,000) annually [17, 18].

In 2010, ~19 % of US adults were smokers. Nationally, a higher percentage of men are smokers than women. Hispanics had a lower prevalence of cigarette smoking than did non-Hispanic whites and African-Americans in the USA in 2010. Among adults in the USA, the prevalence of cigarette smoking generally decreases with age [18].

In both the USA and in Texas, ~20 % of all high school students were current cigarette smokers in 2009. An estimated 5 % of middle school students nationwide and 13 % of middle school students in Texas currently smoke cigarettes [19, 20]. In 2010, an estimated 31 % of all secondary students in Texas reported having used a tobacco product in their lifetime. Even though public health activities have lowered the rate of underage cigarette smoking and tobacco use in Texas considerably since 1990, much still remains to be done [20]. Some factors related to youth tobacco use include low socioeconomic status, parents, guardians, siblings, or peers smoking or approving of tobacco use, accessibility, lack of parental support/involvement, and low self-image or self-esteem [19].

Cigarette Smoking in South Texas

Approximately 17 % of adults in South Texas during 2007–2010 were current smokers. The prevalence of adults who were current smokers in South Texas was slightly but not significantly lower than in the rest of Texas (18.1 %) or nation (18.2 %) (Fig. 8.6).

Sex and age patterns for smoking prevalence in South Texas during 2007–2010 were the same as reported nationwide. Prevalence of current smoking was similar among both Hispanics (17 %) and non-Hispanic whites (16.8 %) in South Texas. Overall, males in South Texas were 1.8 times more likely to be current smokers than females, and among Hispanics, males were 2.5 times more likely than females to be current smokers (Fig. 8.7).

The Lower Rio Grande Valley region had a lower percentage of adults who were current smokers (12.2 %) than South Texas as a whole (16.9 %).

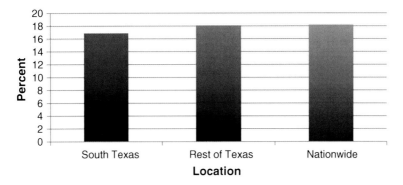

Fig. 8.6 Estimated prevalence of current smoking among adults (18+) by location, 2007–2010. *Source*: Texas Behavioral Risk Factor Surveillance System Combined Year Dataset, Statewide BRFSS Survey, 2007–2010, CDC Behavioral Risk Factor Surveillance System, Nationwide BRFSS Survey, 2007–2010

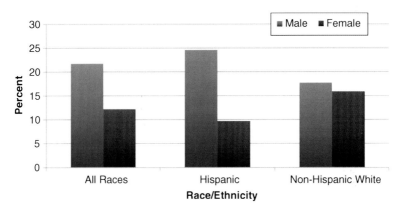

Fig. 8.7 Estimated prevalence of current smoking among South Texas adults by sex and race/ethnicity, 2007–2010. *Source*: Texas Behavioral Risk Factor Surveillance System Combined Year Dataset, Statewide BRFSS Survey, 2007–2010

Alcohol Use

Alcohol is a nervous system depressant that is rapidly absorbed into the blood-stream after consumption. It affects all organs in the body [21]. Excessive alcohol use has both immediate and long-term associated health risks. Possible immediate effects of excessive alcohol use (usually the result of binge drinking) include unintentional injuries, violence, damage to a fetus if pregnant, and alcohol poisoning. Long-term health risks include neurological problems, cardiovascular disease, depression, liver disease, and some cancers. Excessive alcohol use is the third leading lifestyle-related cause of death in the USA, with ~79,000 deaths per year. In 2005, 1.6 million hospitalizations and more than 4 million emergency room visits were alcohol related [22].

When consumed in moderation, alcohol is thought to have some beneficial effects including a reduced risk of cardiovascular disease and all-cause mortality among older adults [14]. However, excessive alcohol use has no benefits whatsoever, and higher morbidity and mortality rates are seen among those who drink large amounts of alcohol [14, 23].

Alcohol use and abuse is more common among males than females, and among younger adults than older ones [22]. Underage drinking is a major public health problem in the USA. Even though alcohol use is illegal for persons under age 21, youth aged 12–20 drink 11 % of all alcohol that is consumed in the USA. It is estimated that more than 40 % of high school students in the USA drink some amount of alcohol. In 2008, 190,000 emergency room visits by persons younger than 21 could be attributed to injuries and other conditions related to alcohol [22].

Heavy Alcohol Consumption

The U.S. Department of Health and Human Services and the U.S. Department of Agriculture's *Dietary Guidelines for Americans* (2010) defines moderate drinking as the consumption of up to one drink a day for women and the consumption of up to two drinks a day for men [14]. Consuming more than one drink per day on average for women or more than two drinks per day on average for men is considered heavy alcohol consumption [22].

Heavy Alcohol Consumption in South Texas

The prevalence of heavy alcohol consumption among adults in South Texas was an estimated 5.5 % in 2007–2010. This prevalence was similar to the percent of heavy alcohol consumption among adults in the rest of Texas (5.0 %) and nation (5.1 %). In South Texas, the prevalence of heavy alcohol consumption was similar between Hispanics (5.4 %) and non-Hispanic whites (5.6 %).

Sex and age patterns for heavy alcohol consumption prevalence in South Texas were the same as observed nationwide. Rates of adult heavy alcohol consumption generally decreased with age (Fig. 8.8), and the prevalence of heavy alcohol consumption was almost twice as high in South Texas males as in females (7.2 % vs. 3.8 %). The prevalence of heavy alcohol consumption was higher, although not statistically significantly higher, in South Texas's metropolitan counties (5.6 %) than in the nonmetropolitan counties (4.1 %).

Binge Drinking

A common pattern of excessive alcohol use in the USA is binge drinking. Binge drinking is defined by the National Institute of Alcohol Abuse and Alcoholism as a

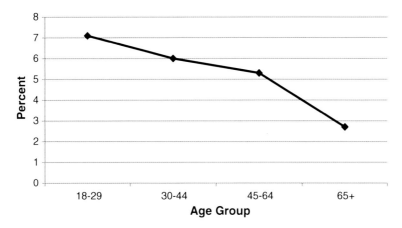

Fig. 8.8 Estimated prevalence of heavy alcohol consumption among South Texas adults by age group, 2007–2010. *Source*: Texas Behavioral Risk Factor Surveillance System Combined Year Dataset, Statewide BRFSS Survey, 2007–2010

pattern of alcohol consumption that brings an individual's blood alcohol concentration (BAC) to 0.08 g percent or greater. For adults, this BAC typically corresponds to drinking five or more drinks in 2 h for males and drinking four or more drinks in 2 h for females [22].

Nationwide, binge drinking is more common among men than women. Binge drinking among underage persons is a problem in the USA. The prevalence of binge drinking in the USA is highest among young adults aged 18–20 (51 %). An estimated one out of every four high school students in the USA binge drink, and more than 90 % of the alcohol consumed by people aged 12–20 is in the form of binge drinks [22].

Binge Drinking in South Texas

In 2007–2010, the prevalence of binge drinking among adults in South Texas was approximately 17.4 %, which was higher than the prevalence for the rest of Texas (14.5 %) and nation (15.1 %). In South Texas, the prevalence of binge drinking was slightly but not statistically significantly higher among Hispanics (18.6 %) than non-Hispanic whites (17.1 %).

The prevalence of binge drinking was much higher for adults aged 18–44 than for adults aged 45 or older. In 2007–2010, approximately one-fourth of all adults aged 18–29 in South Texas binge drank (Fig. 8.9).

The prevalence of binge drinking among South Texas males (25.8 %) was 2.7 times higher than the prevalence among females (9.4 %). The prevalence of binge drinking was higher, though not statistically significantly higher, for South Texas metropolitan county residents (17.9 %) than for residents of nonmetropolitan counties (13.6 %).

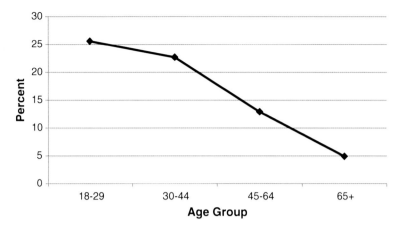

Fig. 8.9 Estimated prevalence of binge drinking among South Texas adults by age group, 2007–2010. *Source*: Texas Behavioral Risk Factor Surveillance System Combined Year Dataset, Statewide BRFSS Survey, 2007–2010

Cancer Screening Activities

Cancer screening is a means of detecting early signs of cancer in people who do not yet have any symptoms. The goal of screening is not to prevent cancer, but rather to find it as early as possible. Positive results obtained from screening tests are not usually diagnostic but can help to identify individuals in whom cancer might be present and thus should be examined further. For some cancers, screening has the potential to reduce deaths and morbidity, because treatment of early-stage cancers often has a better prognosis and can be less aggressive than treatment of advanced-stage cancers [24]. In order for cancer screening to be effective, the test must have the ability to detect cancers earlier than they could be detected as a result of symptoms, and there must be evidence that earlier detection through screening decreases the risk of dying from the disease. Currently, screening tests exist for a number of cancers including breast cancer, cervical cancer, prostate cancer, and colorectal cancer.

Breast Cancer Screening (Mammogram)

Although the breast self-exam and clinical breast exam are also screening methods, the mammogram is currently thought to be the best way to screen for breast cancer [25]. A mammogram is an X-ray of the breast, which can detect tumors that are too small to feel. The capability of a mammogram to detect breast cancer depends on tumor size, breast tissue density, and the skill of the radiologist [26]. Because the incidence of breast cancer increases with age, the Centers for Disease Control and Prevention (CDC) recommend that women aged 50 or older have a mammogram every 2 years [25].

In 2008 and 2010, an estimated 30.5 % of South Texas women aged 40 or older had not had a mammogram in the past 2 years. This estimate was slightly but not significantly higher than the percentage among women in the rest of Texas (28.1 %) during the same time period. However, both South Texas and the rest of Texas had higher percentages of women who had no mammogram in the past 2 years than was seen nationwide (24 %). A slightly but not significantly higher percentage of Hispanic women in South Texas (31.6 %) were estimated to have not had a mammogram in the past 2 years than non-Hispanic whites (28.2 %).

Cervical Cancer Screening (Pap Test)

The Papanicolaou (Pap) test, also called a Pap smear, is the most common screening procedure for cervical cancer. Cells are lightly scraped from the cervix and vagina using a small wooden stick, a brush, or a piece of cotton. The collected cells are then viewed under a microscope to determine if they are normal or abnormal. A Pap test can find the earliest signs of cervical cancer. Because the chance of curing cervical cancer is very high if the cancer is detected early, studies estimate that regular Pap test screening can decrease incidence and mortality of cervical cancer by 80 % or more [27].Doctors recommend Pap tests for women aged 21 or older, or for women under age 21 who have been sexually active for 3 years or more [28, 29].

An estimated 23.3 % of South Texas women aged 18 or older had not had a Pap test in the past 3 years during 2008 and 2010. This South Texas percentage was higher than the percentage of no Pap test in the past 3 years among women in both the rest of Texas (18.3 %) and nation (17.6 %). In South Texas, the percentages of Hispanic and non-Hispanic white women who did not have a Pap test in the past 3 years were similar.

Prostate Cancer Screening

A couple of screening tests for prostate cancer exist: the digital rectal examination (DRE) and the prostate-specific antigen (PSA) test. However, no standard or routine screening is currently recommended for prostate cancer. This is fact that, although these screening tests are able to find prostate cancer at an early stage, not enough evidence currently exists to determine whether early detection and treatment makes any difference in the outcome of the disease [30]. Studies to determine the efficacy of prostate cancer screening are currently underway.

Prostate-Specific Antigen Test

A PSA test measures the amount of PSA in the blood. PSA is a protein made by the prostate gland. Although it is common for men to have low levels of PSA in their

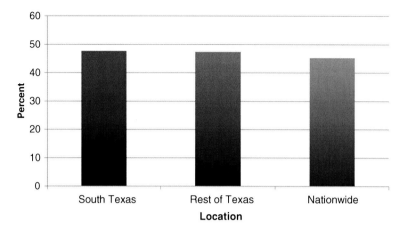

Fig. 8.10 Estimated prevalence of men aged 40 or older who have not had a prostate-specific antigen (PSA) test in the past 2 years by location. *Sources*: Texas data: Texas Behavioral Risk Factor Surveillance System Combined Year Dataset, Statewide BRFSS Survey, 2008, 2010; National data: CDC Behavioral Risk Factor Surveillance System, Nationwide BRFSS Survey data, 2008 and 2010

blood, prostate cancer or other conditions can increase PSA levels. Doctors cannot distinguish between prostate cancer and benign prostate conditions such as inflammation or enlargement of the prostate based on PSA levels alone. However, the PSA test result is taken into account when a doctor makes a decision about whether to do additional tests for prostate cancer. Some doctors encourage PSA tests yearly to screen for prostate cancer, starting anywhere from ages 40–50 [8].

In 2008 and 2010, an estimated 47.7 % of men aged 40 and or older had not had a PSA test in the past 2 years. This was very similar to the prevalence of men aged 40 or older who did not have a PSA test in the past 2 years in the rest of Texas (47.4 %). Estimates for South Texas and the rest of Texas were both slightly but not significantly higher than the nationwide prevalence of not having had a PSA test in the past 2 years (45.3 %) (Fig. 8.10).

In South Texas, Hispanic men were 1.3 times more likely to not have had a PSA test in the past 2 years (54.3 %) than were non-Hispanic white men (41.7 %).

Digital Rectal Exam

DRE is frequently part of a standard physical examination in males. However, it is also another way to screen for prostate cancer and is often performed together with the PSA test to improve the odds of detecting prostate cancer. A doctor performs a digital rectal exam by inserting a lubricated, gloved finger into the rectum to feel the prostate gland through the rectal wall for bumps or anything else abnormal [30, 31].

In 2008 and 2010, an estimated 46 % of men in South Texas had not had a DRE within the past 5 years. This was higher than the prevalence of no DRE within the last 5 years among men in the rest of Texas (38.5 %) and nation (35.6 %). As with PSA testing, Hispanic males in South Texas were more likely to have not had a DRE exam in the past 5 years (57.5 %) than were non-Hispanic white males (33.9 %).

Colorectal Cancer Screening

Several tests are regularly used to screen for colorectal cancer, including the fetal occult blood test (FOBT), sigmoidoscopy, colonoscopy, the double-contrast barium enema (DCBE), and newer techniques such as virtual colonoscopy [32]. Based on several studies, the U.S. Preventive Services Task Force (USPSTF) found evidence that FOBT, sigmoidoscopy, and colonoscopy screening methods are effective in reducing colorectal cancer mortality, and recommends screening using any of these methods for adults aged 50–75 [33].

Fecal Occult Blood Testing

FOBT is a frequently used noninvasive colorectal cancer screening option that checks for hidden blood in the stool. Stool samples are collected at home, placed on special cards, and are then given back to a doctor or lab for testing. Blood in the stool can be indicative of polyps or cancer [32]. Studies have found that for persons aged 50–80, having an annual or biennial FOBT may reduce colorectal cancer mortality by up to 33 % [34]. One of the recommended American Cancer Society colorectal cancer testing options is an annual FOBT for persons aged 50 or older [35].

An estimated 83.9 % of individuals aged 50 or older in South Texas had not had a FOBT in the past 2 years in 2008 and 2010. This South Texas prevalence was similar to the prevalence of no FOBT in the rest of Texas (82.7 %) but was significantly higher than the prevalence seen nationwide (80 %). In South Texas, Hispanics had a higher prevalence of not having an FOBT within the past 2 years (87.5 %) than non-Hispanic whites (81 %).

Sigmoidoscopy/Colonoscopy

Sigmoidoscopy and colonoscopy are two other common colon cancer screening procedures. Sigmoidoscopy checks the rectum and *lower* colon by inserting a thin, flexible, lighted instrument in through the rectum. A colonoscopy is an examination of the rectum and *whole* colon for polyps, cancer, or other abnormalities using a similar thin, lighted instrument [32, 34]. Both sigmoidoscopy and colonoscopy procedures have higher sensitivity than FOBT, and colonoscopy is the most sensitive and specific colorectal cancer test [33]. However, unlike FOBT, sigmoidoscopy and colonoscopy are both invasive procedures, and colonoscopy in particular has associated risks such as bleeding or perforation of the colon [33, 34]. Recommended American Cancer Society colorectal cancer testing options for those older than 50 include either a sigmoidoscopy every 5 years, a yearly FOBT, or a colonoscopy every 10 years [35].

In South Texas, an estimated 42.8 % of individuals older than 50 had never had a sigmoidoscopy or colonoscopy in 2008 and 2010. This prevalence was slightly but not significantly higher than the prevalence seen in the rest of Texas (40.2 %) and was statistically significantly higher than the prevalence of no sigmoidoscopy or colonoscopy observed nationwide (35.9 %). As with the prevalence of no FOBT screening, a higher percentage of Hispanics older than 50 in South Texas had never had a sigmoidoscopy or colonoscopy (52.6 %) than non-Hispanic whites (32.4 %).

Summary

Table 8.1 Summary table of adult behavioral risk factor prevalences in South Texas, the rest of Texas, and nationwide

Health indicator	Prevalence (%)[a]		
	South Texas	Rest of Texas	Nationwide
Obesity	32.7	29.1	27.0
Inadequate physical activity	51.8	52.4	51.1
Inadequate fruit and vegetable consumption	76.2	75.1	75.8
Current cigarette smoking	16.9	18.1	18.2
Heavy alcohol consumption	5.5	5.0	5.1
Binge drinking	17.4	14.5	15.1
Had no mammogram in past 2 years (women)	30.5	28.1	24.0
Had no Pap test in past 2 years (women)	23.3	18.3	17.6
Had no PSA test in past 2 years (men)	47.7	47.4	45.3
Had no digital rectal exam in past 2 years (men)	46.0	38.5	35.6
Had no blood stool test in past 2 years	83.9	82.7	80.0
Never had a sigmoidoscopy/colonoscopy	42.8	40.2	35.9

[a]Texas data were obtained from a Texas Behavioral Risk Factor Surveillance System (BRFSS) Combined Year Dataset of the statewide BRFSS survey, and all nationwide estimates were calculated using national BRFSS combined year survey data. For both Texas and nationwide estimates, obesity, current cigarette smoking, heavy alcohol consumption, binge drinking, and current asthma prevalence estimates were calculated using 2007–2010 survey data, all cancer screening test prevalences were calculated using 2008 and 2010 survey data, and inadequate physical activity and inadequate fruit and vegetable consumption used 2007 and 2009 survey data

References

1. Ogden C, Carroll M, Kit B, Flegal K. Prevalence of obesity in the United States, 2009–2010. NCHS Data Brief. 2012;82:1–7.
2. Centers for Disease Control and Prevention. Childhood overweight and obesity. 2012. http://www.cdc.gov/obesity/childhood/index.html. Accessed May 2012.
3. Centers for Disease Control and Prevention. Adult obesity facts. 2012. http://www.cdc.gov/obesity/data/adult.html. Accessed May 2012.
4. Arons A. Childhood obesity in Texas: the costs, the policies, and a framework for the future. 2011. http://www.childhealthtx.org/pdfs/Childhood%20Obesity%20in%20Texas%20Report.pdf. Accessed May 2012.
5. National Conference of State Legislatures. Childhood overweight and obesity trends. 2012. http://www.ncsl.org/issues-research/health/childhood-obesity-trends-state-rates.aspx. Accessed May 2012.
6. Freedman DS, Khan LK, Serdula MK, Dietz WH, Srinivasan SR, Berenson GS. The relation of childhood BMI to adult adiposity: the Bogalusa heart study. Pediatrics. 2005;115:22–7.
7. National Collaborative on Childhood Obesity Research. Childhood obesity in the United States. 2009. http://www.nccor.org/downloads/ChildhoodObesity_020509.pdf. Accessed May 2012.
8. Texas Department of State Health Services. The burden of overweight and obesity in Texas, 2000–2040. 2003. http://www.dshs.state.tx.us/obesity/pdf/Cost_Obesity_Report.pdf. Accessed May 2013.
9. Centers for Disease Control and Prevention. Overweight and obesity. 2012. http://www.cdc.gov/obesity/adult/index.html. Accessed May 2012.
10. U.S. Department of Health and Human Services. 2008 Physical activity guidelines for Americans. 2008. http://www.health.gov/paguidelines/pdf/paguide.pdf. Accessed June 2012.
11. Centers for Disease Control and Prevention. Physical activity for everyone: recommendations. 2011. http://www.cdc.gov/nccdphp/dnpa/physical/recommendations/index.htm. Accessed June 2012
12. Centers for Disease Control and Prevention. Physical activity and good nutrition: essential elements to prevent chronic diseases and obesity, 2008. CS117151. U.S. Department of Health and Human Services, Centers for Disease Control and Prevention; 2008.
13. Centers for Disease Control and Prevention. Fruits and veggies matter: fruit and vegetable benefits. 2007. http://www.fruitsandveggiesmatter.gov/benefits/index.html. . Accessed June 2012.
14. U.S. Department of Agriculture and U.S. Department of Health and Human Services. Dietary guidelines for Americans, 2010. 7th ed. Washington, DC: U.S. Government Printing Office; 2010.
15. Centers for Disease Control and Prevention. Fruit and vegetable consumption data and statistics. 2009. Accessed June 2012.
16. Centers for Disease Control and Prevention. Fact sheet: health effects of cigarette smoking. 2012. http://www.cdc.gov/tobacco/data_statistics/fact_sheets/health_effects/effects_cig_smoking/index.htm. Accessed June 2012.
17. Adhikari B, Kahende J, Malarcher A, Pechacek T, Tong V. Smoking-attributable mortality, years of potential life lost, and productivity losses – United States, 2000–2004. MMWR. 2008;57:1226–8.
18. Centers for Disease Control and Prevention. Fact sheet – adult cigarette smoking in the United States: current estimates. 2012. http://www.cdc.gov/tobacco/data_statistics/fact_sheets/adult_data/cig_smoking/index.htm. Accessed June 2012.
19. Centers for Disease Control and Prevention. Fact sheet – youth and tobacco use: current estimates. 2012. http://www.cdc.gov/tobacco/data_statistics/fact_sheets/youth_data/tobacco_use/index.htm. Accessed June 2012.

20. Texas Department of State Health Services. Texans and tobacco: report to the 82nd Texas legislature. 2011. http://www.dshs.state.tx.us/WorkArea/linkit.aspx?LinkIdentifier= id&ItemID=8589952884. Accessed May 2013.
21. Centers for Disease Control and Prevention. Alcohol and public health: frequently asked questions. 2012. http://www.cdc.gov/alcohol/faqs.htm. Accessed June 2012.
22. Alcohol and Public Health fact sheets. 2010. http://www.cdc.gov/alcohol/fact-sheets.htm. Accessed June 2012.
23. Goldberg RJ, Burchfiel CM, Reed DM, Wergowske G, Chiu D. A prospective study of the health effects of health effects of alcohol consumption in middle-aged and elderly men: the Honolulu Heart Program. Circulation. 1994;89:651–9.
24. National Cancer Institute. Cancer screening overview. 2012. http://www.cancer.gov/cancertopics/pdq/screening/overview/. Accessed June 2012.
25. Centers for Disease Control and Prevention. Breast cancer – screening. 2012. http://www.cdc.gov/cancer/breast/basic_info/screening.htm. Accessed June 2012.
26. National Cancer Institute. Breast cancer screening. 2011. http://www.cancer.gov/cancertopics/pdq/screening/breast/. Accessed June 2012.
27. National Cancer Institute. Cervical cancer screening. 2012. http://www.cancer.gov/cancertopics/pdq/screening/cervical/. Accessed June 2012.
28. National Women's Health Information Center. Pap test – frequently asked questions. U.S. Department of Health and Human Services, Office on Women's Health. 2009.
29. Centers for Disease Control and Prevention. Gynecologic cancers – cervical cancer screening. 2012. http://www.cdc.gov/cancer/cervical/basic_info/screening.htm. Accessed June 2012.
30. National Cancer Institute. Prostate cancer screening. 2012. http://www.cancer.gov/cancertopics/pdq/screening/prostate/. Accessed June 2012.
31. National Cancer Institute. National Cancer Institute factsheet: prostate-specific antigen (PSA) test. 2009. http://www.cancer.gov/cancertopics/factsheet/Detection/PSA. Accessed June 2012.
32. National Cancer Institute. Colorectal cancer screening. 2011. http://www.cancer.gov/cancertopics/pdq/screening/colorectal/. Accessed June 2012.
33. U.S. Preventive Services Task Force. Screening for colorectal cancer: U.S. preventive services task force recommendation statement. Ann Intern Med. 2008;149:627–37.
34. National Cancer Institute. National Cancer Institute factsheet: colorectal cancer screening. 2011. http://www.cancer.gov/cancertopics/factsheet/Detection/colorectal-screening. Accessed June 2012.
35. American Cancer Society. American Cancer Society guidelines for the early detection of cancer. 2012. http://www.cancer.org/docroot/ped/content/ped_2_3x_acs_cancer_detection_guidelines_36.asp. Accessed June 2012.

Chapter 9
Environmental Health Issues

A broad range of different environmental exposures can cause health problems including air and water pollution, exposure to lead and other heavy metals, pesticides and chemicals, and many more. This chapter covers two main environmental exposure health status indicators: elevated child blood lead levels and pesticide exposures.

Childhood Lead Poisoning

Lead is a significant and widespread environmental hazard for all Texas children. Exposure to lead can lead to a number of medical conditions including long-term neurological damage that is often associated with learning and behavioral problems. Blood lead levels ≥10 µg/dL are considered to be elevated, although a child may often not show symptoms, even at higher levels. Very elevated lead levels can result in death. Lead is a ubiquitous toxin with varied exposure sources including dust or chips from lead-based paints, contaminated soil, crafts/hobbies, and home remedy/folk medicines.

With increased awareness and efforts to reduce exposure, childhood lead poisoning has decreased in recent years. In 2005, 54,051 US children aged 6 or younger tested with confirmed elevated blood lead levels, compared to 24,375 children in 2009, a decrease of 55 % in 5 years [1]. Children aged 6 or younger are at greater risk of lead poisoning than older children due to increased absorption, predominant hand-to-mouth behavior, and developing neurological systems. Among US children younger than 6 in 1999–2004, African-American children had a higher percentage of elevated blood lead levels (3.4 %) than did Hispanic children (1.2 %) or non-Hispanic white children (1.2 %) [2]. Children who live or spend a significant amount of time in pre-1950s housing are at increased risk of childhood lead poisoning. Poverty and living in an area of existing high childhood lead prevalence are also considered surrogate markers for a child's potential lead exposure risk.

A.G. Ramirez et al. (eds.), *The South Texas Health Status Review:*
A Health Disparities Roadmap, DOI 10.1007/978-3-319-00233-0_9, © The Author(s) 2013

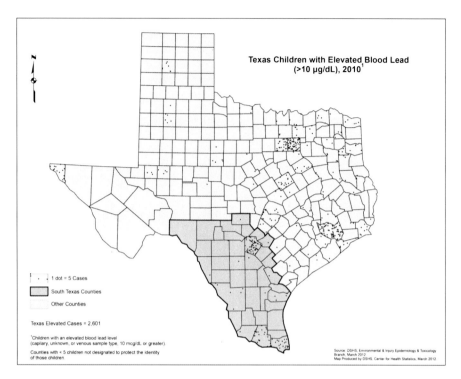

Fig. 9.1 Texas children aged 0–14 with elevated blood lead levels (≥10 µg/dL) by location of residence, 2010. *Source*: Texas Childhood Lead Poisoning Prevention Program, Texas Department of State Health Services

Childhood Lead Poisoning in South Texas

In terms of sheer numbers, Bexar County and the Lower Rio Grande Valley region had the most children aged 0–14 with elevated blood lead levels (>10 µg/dL) in South Texas (Fig. 9.1). Numbers are most likely greater in these areas because of relatively large population sizes or because of a large percentage of people with low socioeconomic status living in the area.

Overall, the percent of children aged 0–14 with elevated blood lead levels among those tested in South Texas was 0.9 %, a slightly higher percentage than among those tested in the rest of Texas (0.8 %) (Fig. 9.2). However, for non-Hispanic white children, the percentage with elevated blood lead levels of those tested was lower in South Texas (0.4 %) than in the rest of Texas (1.2 %). In South Texas, among Hispanic children tested, 1.2 % had elevated blood lead levels, whereas among non-Hispanic white children tested, only 0.4 % had elevated blood lead levels (Fig. 9.2).

In South Texas, for both Hispanic and non-Hispanic white children, the youngest age group (aged 0–2) had the highest percent of elevated blood lead levels among those tested (Fig. 9.3). However, for all three age groups, Hispanic children in South Texas had higher percentages of elevated lead levels among those tested than did non-Hispanic white children in South Texas (Fig. 9.3).

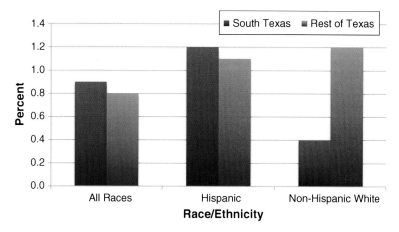

Fig. 9.2 Percent of South Texas children 0–14 years of age with elevated blood lead levels (≥10 µg/dL) among children tested, 2006–2010. *Source*: Texas Childhood Lead Poisoning Prevention Program,Texas Department of State Health Services

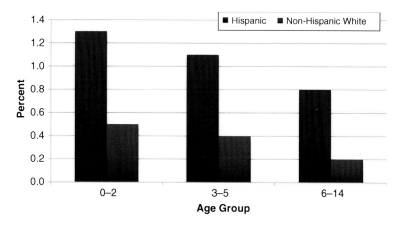

Fig. 9.3 Percent of South Texas children aged 0–14 with elevated blood lead levels (≥10 µg/dL) among children tested, by age group and race/ethnicity, 2006–2010. *Source*: Texas Childhood Lead Poisoning Prevention Program, Texas Department of State Health Services

In South Texas, the percentage of boys with elevated blood lead levels among those tested (1.0 %) was slightly higher than the percentage of girls with elevated blood lead levels (0.8 %). The percentage of children with elevated blood lead levels (of those tested) was similar between nonmetropolitan South Texas counties (1.0 %) and metropolitan counties (0.9 %).

The percent of elevated blood lead levels among children tested was slightly but not significantly higher in Webb County (1.2 %) than in South Texas as a whole (0.9 %). The percentage of children with elevated blood lead levels was the same in the Lower Rio Grande Valley region and Bexar County (0.9 %) as in South Texas (Fig. 9.4).

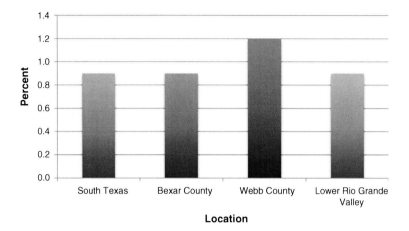

Fig. 9.4 Percent of children aged 0–14 with elevated blood lead levels ($\geq$10 μg/dL) among children tested in selected South Texas locations, 2006–2010. *Source*: Texas Childhood Lead Poisoning Prevention Program, Texas Department of State Health Services

Work-Related Pesticide Exposure

A pesticide is any substance or combination of substances that is used for preventing, repelling, controlling, or destroying any type of pest. Types of pesticides include not only insecticides but also herbicides, fungicides, rodenticides, disinfectants, and sanitizers [3]. In the USA, about 1.1 billion pounds of pesticide active ingredient are used each year, and more than 20,000 different pesticide products are currently sold nationwide [4]. Although pesticides are useful to society, they also have the potential to cause great harm to humans, because they are designed to kill or damage living organisms. Health effects vary depending on the type of pesticide involved and the level of exposure. Acute high-level pesticide exposures can cause nausea and vomiting, skin or eye irritation, difficulty breathing, seizures, or even death [5]. Long-term pesticide exposure effects have been associated with changes in neurobehavioral performance, neurological damage and diseases [6, 7], and certain types of cancers [8]. Children are particularly susceptible to pesticides [9].

Acute pesticide exposures are most commonly occupational exposures. In 2008, the annual rate of work-related pesticide poisonings in the USA was estimated to be 1.5 per 100,000 workers. [10] Agricultural workers are at especially high risk of pesticide exposure. The annual incidence of pesticide-related illness among agricultural workers from 1998 to 2007 time period was approximately 48/100,000 [11]. This high incidence among persons employed in agriculture is of particular concern for Hispanics, because 88 % of all farm workers in the USA are Hispanic. Because of pesticide drift, people who live in agricultural areas have a higher risk of pesticide exposure than people who live in nonagricultural areas [9]. For all occupations

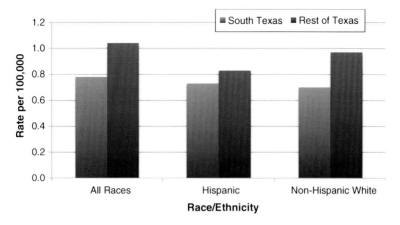

Fig. 9.5 Incidence of work-related pesticide exposure by location and race/ethnicity, 2006–2010. *Source*: Pesticide Exposure Surveillance in Texas (PEST) program, Texas Department of State Health Services

combined, males have a slightly higher risk of pesticide-related illness than do females; however, among agricultural workers, the incidence of pesticide-related illness in females is higher than the incidence in males [11, 12].

Work-Related Pesticide Exposure in South Texas

Overall, the South Texas working population had a slightly lower incidence of pesticide exposure (0.8 cases per 100,000 population) than did workers in the rest of Texas (1.0/100,000). Hispanics in South Texas had an incidence of pesticide exposure (0.7/100,000) that was comparable to the incidence for Hispanics in the rest of Texas (0.8/100,000) (Fig. 9.5). In South Texas, the incidence of pesticide exposure was similar between Hispanics and non-Hispanic whites (0.7/100,000); however, in the rest of Texas, incidence was slightly but not significantly higher for non-Hispanic whites (1.0/100,000) than for Hispanics (0.8/100,000) (Fig. 9.5).

In South Texas, the incidence of occupational pesticide exposure was slightly but not significantly higher in males (0.9/100,000) than females (0.6/100,000). Residents of nonmetropolitan counties in South Texas had a significantly higher incidence of occupational pesticide exposure (2.2/100,000) than did those in metropolitan counties (1.3/100,000). Adults aged 20–59 had higher incidences of work-related pesticide exposure than other age groups (Fig. 9.6).

From 2006 to 2010, incidences of work-related pesticide exposure in Bexar County (0.7/100,000) and the Lower Rio Grande Valley (0.8/100,000) were comparable to the incidence seen in South Texas as a whole (0.8/100,000). The incidence of work-related pesticide exposure in Webb County could not be compared, as the number of cases over this time period was too few to report (Fig. 9.7).

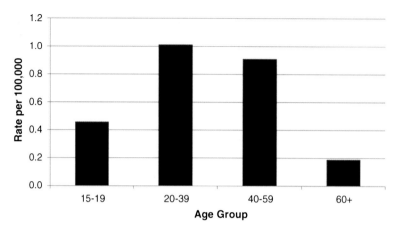

Fig. 9.6 Incidence of work-related pesticide exposure in South Texas by age group, 2006–2010. *Source*: Pesticides Exposure Surveillance in Texas (PEST) program, Texas Department of State Health Services

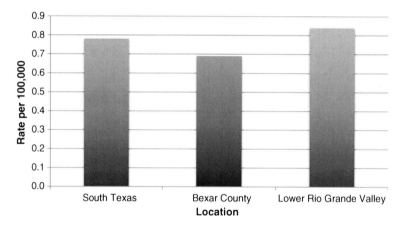

Fig. 9.7 Incidence of work-related pesticide exposure in selected South Texas locations, 2006–2010. No rate is shown for Webb County because the number of cases in this county was too few to report. *Source*: Pesticides Exposure Surveillance in Texas (PEST) program, Texas Department of State Health Services

Summary

Table 9.1 Summary table of estimates in South Texas, the rest of Texas, and nationwide[a] for each of the environmental health indicators analyzed

Health indicator	Incidence/prevalence estimates		
	South Texas, 2006–2010	Rest of Texas, 2006–2010	Nationwide
Childhood lead poisoning	0.9 % of those tested	0.8 % of those tested	[b]

[a]Nationwide estimates were not available for all health indicators in the table
[b]Signifies that no nationwide estimate could be found for the health indicator

References

1. Centers for Disease Control and Prevention. Number of children tested and confirmed EBLLs by state, year, and BLL group, children <72 months old. 2009. http://www.cdc.gov/nceh/lead/data/StateConfirmedByYear_1997_2009.htm. Accessed May 2012.
2. Jones RL, Homa DM, Meyer PA, Brody DJ, Caldwell KL, Pirkle JL, et al. Trends in blood lead levels and blood lead testing among US children aged 1 to 5 years, 1999–2004. Pediatrics. 2009;123:e376–85.
3. U S Environmental Protection Agency. About pesticides: what is a pesticide? 2006. http://www.epa.gov/pesticides/about/index.htm. Accessed May 2007.
4. National Institute for Occupational Safety and Health, Centers for Disease Control and Prevention. Pesticide illness and injury surveillance. 2011. http://www.cdc.gov/niosh/topics/pesticides/. Accessed May 2012.
5. The Mid-Atlantic Center for Children's Health and the Environment. Pesticides. 2003. http://www.childrensnational.org/MACCHE/ResourcesAndTutorials/Pesticides.aspx. Accessed May 2007.
6. Rothlein J, Rohlman D, Lasarev M, Phillips J, Muniz J, McCauley L. Organophosphate pesticide exposure and neurobehavioral performance in agricultural and non-agricultural Hispanic workers. Environ Health Perspect. 2006;114:691–6.
7. Kamel F, Hoppin JA. Association of pesticide exposure with neurologic dysfunction and disease. Environ Health Perspect. 2004;112:950–8.
8. National Cancer Institute. Cancer trends progress report – 2009/2010 update. 2007. http://progressreport.cancer.gov/doc_detail.asp?pid=1&did=2009&chid=91&coid=913&mid=. Accessed Apr 2012.
9. Quintero-Somaini A, Quirindongo M, Arevalo E, Lashof D, Olson E, Solomon G. Hidden danger: environmental health threats in the latino community. National Resources Defense Council; 2004.
10. Council of State and Territorial Epidemiologists. Indicator 11: acute work-related pesticide poisonings reported to poison control centers. 2011. http://www.cste.org/dnn/ProgramsandActivities/OccupationalHealth/OccupationalHealthIndicators/Indicator11/tabid/107/Default.aspx. Accessed May 2012.
11. Kasner EJ, Keralis JM, Mehler L, Beckman J, Bonnar-Prado J, Lee S-J, et al. Gender differences in acute pesticide-related illnesses and injuries among farmworkers in the United States, 1998–2007. Am J Ind Med. 2012;55(7):571–83.
12. Calvert GM, Plate DK, Das R, Rosales R, Shafey O, Thomsen C, et al. Acute occupational pesticide-related illness in the U.S., 1998–1999: surveillance findings from SENSOR-pesticides program. Am J Ind Med. 2004;45:14–23.

Chapter 10
Injury

Injury is a significant public health problem in the USA, causing disability and premature death regardless of race, sex, or economic status and creating a tremendous burden on our national health care system [1]. Injury is the leading cause of both disability and death in American children and young adults and is the fifth-leading cause of death overall in the USA [1, 2]. An estimated 182,479 individuals in the USA died from injuries in 2007 [1]. In 2007, more than 29 million people were treated for injuries in hospital emergency departments in America, and 2.8 million of these injuries were so severe that they required hospitalization [1]. Even though there are many types of injuries that contribute to injury mortality, three of the leading causes of death by injury in the USA are motor vehicle crashes, suicide, and homicide [1]. Mortality due to injuries is presented as age-adjusted rates.

Motor Vehicle Crash Mortality

A motor vehicle crash (MVC) is any collision involving one or more ground-transportation motor vehicles. MVCs are the leading cause of injury death in the USA and are the leading cause of death overall among persons aged 5–34 [1, 2]. MVCs accounted for more than 33,800 US deaths in 2009 [3]. It is estimated that an additional 2.3 million persons suffer from nonfatal injuries associated with MVCs each year [3, 4].

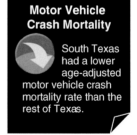

Motor Vehicle Crash Mortality

South Texas had a lower age-adjusted motor vehicle crash mortality rate than the rest of Texas.

Nationwide, men have a higher MVC mortality rate than women [5]. The risk of MVC mortality is higher among teen drivers (aged 16–19) and drivers aged 80 and older than among the other age groups in the USA [6]. In 2009, MVC mortality rates were 12.1 per 100,000 population for non-Hispanic whites, 10.4/100,000 for Hispanics, and 12.0/100,000 for African-Americans in the USA [7]. Other risk factors for motor

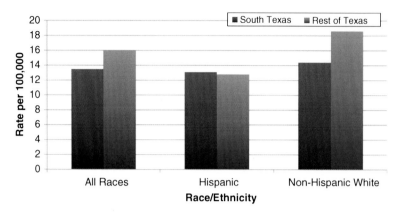

Fig. 10.1 Motor vehicle crash (MVC) mortality rates by location and race/ethnicity, 2005–2009. *Source*: Center for Health Statistics Data Management Team, Texas Department of State Health Services

vehicle-related fatalities include alcohol or other drug use and not wearing a seat belt [6]. In 2009, nearly one-third of all MVC-related fatalities occurring in the USA involved alcohol [8].

Motor Vehicle Crash Mortality in South Texas

Overall, South Texas had a lower age-adjusted motor vehicle crash mortality rate (13.5/100,000) than the rest of Texas (16.0/100,000) in 2005–2009. Although non-Hispanic whites in South Texas had a lower MVC mortality rate compared with non-Hispanic whites in the rest of Texas, rates were similar between Hispanics in South Texas and Hispanics in the rest of Texas (Fig. 10.1).

The highest MVC mortality rates in South Texas were observed among individuals aged 15–24 (20.7/100,000) and those aged 75 and older (20.9/100,000). The MVC mortality rate for South Texas males (19.4/100,000) was 2.5 times higher than the mortality rate for females (7.9/100,000). Residents of nonmetropolitan counties in South Texas had a higher MVC mortality rate (19.6/100,000) than did residents of metropolitan counties (12.6/100,000). Mortality rates in Bexar County (12.5/100,000), Webb County (12.1/100,000), and the Lower Rio Grande Valley area (12.2/100,000) were not significantly different than the MVC mortality rate in South Texas as a whole (13.5/100,000).

Homicide Mortality

The International Classification of Diseases, 10th Revision, defines homicide as any intentional injury inflicted by another person with the intent to kill [9]. Homicide, especially among young people, is a serious US public health issue [10]. In 2007,

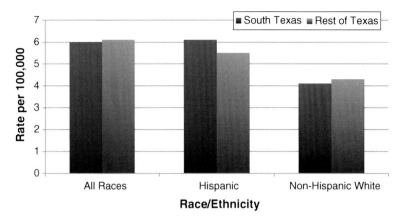

Fig. 10.2 Homicide mortality rates by location and race/ethnicity, 2005–2009. *Source*: Center for Health Statistics Data Management Team, Texas Department of State Health Services

homicide was the second-leading cause of death nationwide in young adults aged 10–24 [11] and was the third-leading cause of death among adults aged 25–34 [12]. In 2007, more than 18,000 homicide deaths were reported in the USA [10], and more than 5,700 of these homicide victims were aged 10–24 [11].

Nationwide, males are more than 3.5 times more likely to die from homicide than females. African-Americans were more than seven times more likely to be murdered than non-Hispanic whites in 2007, and Hispanics also had a higher homicide rate than non-Hispanic whites [13, 14]. US homicide rates are highest among young adults aged 20–24. However, among persons younger than 18, a "U"-shaped trend in homicide is seen, with infants having a significantly higher homicide rate (3.6/100,000) than those aged 5–9 (0.7/100,000) and 10–14 (1.0/100,000) [14]. Other risk factors associated with homicide include living in urban areas, low socioeconomic status, and access to firearms [13, 14].

Homicide Mortality in South Texas

Overall, the age-adjusted homicide rate in South Texas (6.0/100,000) was very similar to rates in the rest of Texas (6.1/100,000) and nationwide (6.0/100,000) [7]. In South Texas, a higher rate of homicide was observed among Hispanics (6.1/100,000) than among non-Hispanic whites (4.1/100,000) (Fig. 10.2). Among Hispanics, homicide rates in South Texas (6.1/100,000) were slightly higher than in the rest of Texas (5.5/100,000).

In South Texas, homicide rates were highest among individuals aged 15–24 (9.3/100,000) and aged 25–34 (11.2/100,000). Overall, males in South Texas were more than three times more likely to be murdered than females, and among Hispanics, males were four times more likely to be murdered. The homicide rate difference between the two sexes was much smaller for non-Hispanic whites (Fig. 10.3).

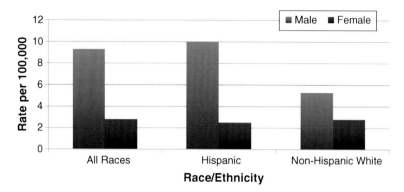

Fig. 10.3 Homicide mortality rates in South Texas by sex and race/ethnicity, 2005–2009. *Source*: Center for Health Statistics Data Management Team, Texas Department of State Health Services.

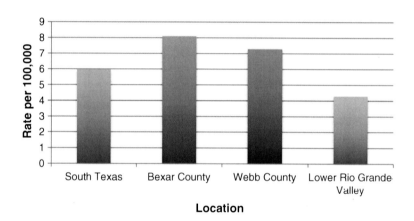

Fig. 10.4 Homicide mortality rates in selected South Texas locations, 2005–2009. *Source*: Center for Health Statistics Data Management Team, Texas Department of State Health Services

A higher homicide rate was seen in Bexar County than in South Texas as a whole, while the Lower Rio Grande Valley area had a lower homicide rate than all of South Texas (Fig. 10.4). There were a sufficient number of homicide cases within Bexar County to stratify these cases by race/ethnicity. In Bexar County, the homicide rate was four times higher among African-Americans (21.0/100,000) and more than 1.5 times higher among Hispanics (8.4/100,000) than among non-Hispanic whites (5.0/100,000) (Fig. 10.5).

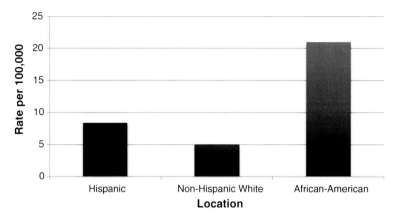

Fig. 10.5 Homicide mortality rates in Bexar County by race/ethnicity, 2005–2009. *Source:* Center for Health Statistics Data Management Team, Texas Department of State Health Services

Suicide Mortality

Suicide is the intentional act of taking one's own life. Suicide is the tenth leading cause of death overall in the USA [15], is the second leading cause of death among adults age 25 to 34, and is the third leading cause of death among persons 15–24 years of age [2, 15]. Suicide was responsible for more than 36,000 deaths in the USA in 2009 [7, 15]. In 2007, 4,140 young adults ages 15–24 completed a suicide [2]. However, suicide mortality only indicates a small portion of the amount of suicidal behaviors taking place in the USA. Among young adults 15–24 years old, there are between 100 and 200 attempts of suicide for every completed act [16]. Firearms are used in the majority of suicide deaths in the USA [13, 15].

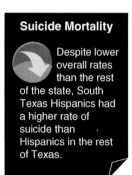

Suicide Mortality

Despite lower overall rates than the rest of the state, South Texas Hispanics had a higher rate of suicide than Hispanics in the rest of Texas.

While women are more likely to think about and to attempt suicide, males are nearly four times more likely to die from suicide [16]. In fact, suicide was the seventh-leading cause of death among US males in 2007, and almost 80 % of all suicide deaths occur in males [2, 16]. In 2009, US suicide rates were highest among persons aged 40–59 [7], and higher rates have also been observed among the elderly [15, 16]. Nationwide, non-Hispanic whites have higher suicide rates than all other race/ethnic groups [7]. Risk factors for suicide include previous attempts at suicide, a history of depression, easy access to lethal methods, alcohol or drug abuse, physical illness, and feelings of isolation [17].

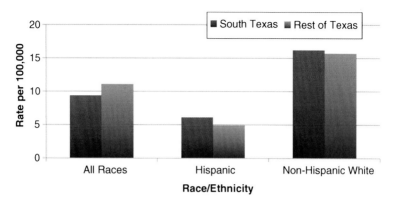

Fig. 10.6 Suicide mortality rates by location and race/ethnicity, 2005–2009. *Source*: Center for Health Statistics Data Management Team, Texas Department of State Health Services

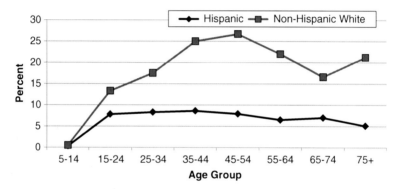

Fig. 10.7 Suicide mortality rates in South Texas by age group and race/ethnicity, 2005–2009. *Source*: Center for Health Statistics Data Management Team, Texas Department of State Health Services

Suicide Mortality in South Texas

Overall, South Texas had a lower age-adjusted suicide rate (9.4/100,000) during 2005–2009 than observed in the rest of Texas (11.1/100,000) or nationwide (11.3/100,000) [7]. However, Hispanics in South Texas had a higher rate of suicide than Hispanics in the rest of Texas (6.1/100,000 vs. 4.9/100,000). In both South Texas and the rest of Texas, suicide rates were between 2.5 and 3.2 times higher among non-Hispanic whites than among Hispanics (Fig. 10.6).

In South Texas, suicide rates were higher among non-Hispanic whites than among Hispanics for individuals aged 15 and older. For non-Hispanic whites in South Texas, suicide rates were highest among the 35–44 and 45–54 age groups, declined among individuals aged 55–74, and then increased again among the oldest age group. For Hispanics, however, suicide rates remained much the same among individuals older than 15 (Fig. 10.7).

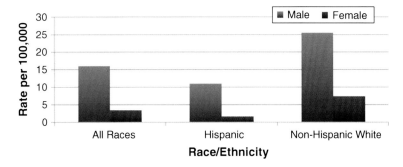

Fig. 10.8 Suicide mortality rates in South Texas by sex and race/ethnicity, 2005–2009. *Source*: Center for Health Statistics Data Management Team, Texas Department of State Health Services

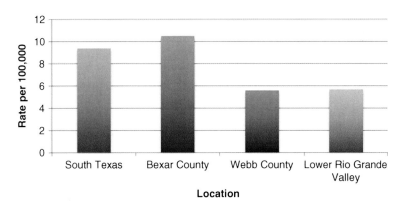

Fig. 10.9 Suicide mortality rates in selected South Texas locations, 2005–2009. *Source*: Center for Health Statistics Data Management Team, Texas Department of State Health Services

Overall, the suicide rate among South Texas males was almost five times higher than among females. Among Hispanics, the risk of suicide death was almost seven times higher in males than in females, and among non-Hispanic whites, males were almost 3.5 times more likely to die of suicide (Fig. 10.8). As observed nationwide, non-Hispanic white males in South Texas are at the highest risk for suicide mortality. The age-adjusted suicide rate among non-Hispanic white males in South Texas was 25.5/100,000 (Fig. 10.8).

The suicide rate in Bexar County (10.5/100,000) was slightly higher than in South Texas as a whole (9.4/100,000); however, suicide rates in Webb County (5.6/100,000) and the Lower Rio Grande Valley region (5.7/100,000) were both significantly lower than in South Texas (Fig. 10.9).

Summary

Table 10.1 Summary table of age-adjusted mortality rates in South Texas, the rest of Texas, and nationwide[a] for each of the injury health indicators analyzed

| Health indicator | Mortality rate per 100,000 population | | |
	South Texas, 2005–2009	Rest of Texas, 2005–2009	Nationwide, 2005–2009
Motor vehicle crash mortality	13.5	16.0	[b]
Homicide	6.0	6.1	6.0
Suicide	9.4	11.1	11.3

[a]Nationwide estimates were not available for all health indicators in the table
[b]Signifies that no nationwide mortality rate could be found for the health indicator

References

1. Centers for Disease Control and Prevention. Injury prevention and control. 2012. http://www.cdc.gov/injury/overview/. Accessed May 2012.
2. Centers for Disease Control and Prevention. WISQARS leading causes of death reports, 1999–2007. 2010. http://webappa.cdc.gov/sasweb/ncipc/leadcaus10.html. Accessed May 2012.
3. National Highway Traffic Safety Administration. Traffic safety facts: highlights of 2009 motor vehicle crashes. Washington, DC: U.S. Department of Transportation; 2010.
4. Beck L, West B. Vital signs: nonfatal, motor vehicle–occupant injuries (2009) and seat belt use (2008) among adults–United States. MMWR. 2011;59:1681–6.
5. Ingram DD, Franco SJ. QuickStats: age-adjusted motor vehicle accident death rates, by sex and type of locality – United States, 2007–2009. MMWR. 2012,61:197.
6. Centers for Disease Control and Prevention. Injury prevention and control: motor vehicle safety. 2011. http://www.cdc.gov/motorvehiclesafety/index.html. Accessed May 2012.
7. Centers for Disease Control and Prevention. WISQARS fatal injury reports, national and regional, 1999–2009. 2010. http://webappa.cdc.gov/sasweb/ncipc/mortrate10_us.html. Accessed May 2012.
8. Bergen G, Shults R, Rudd R. Vital signs: alcohol-impaired driving among adults–United States, 2010. MMWR. 2011;60:1351–6.
9. World Health Organization. International statistical classification of diseases and related health problems, 10th Revision. France: World Health Organization; 1992.
10. Centers for Disease Control and Prevention. Injury Center – violence prevention. 2012. http://www.cdc.gov/violenceprevention/. Accessed May 2012.
11. Centers for Disease Control and Prevention, National Center for Injury Prevention and Control. Youth violence: facts at a glance. 2010. http://www.cdc.gov/ViolencePrevention/pdf/YV-DataSheet-a.pdf. Accessed May 2012.
12. Centers for Disease Control and Prevention. WISQARS leading causes of death reports, 2007. 2010. http://webappa.cdc.gov/sasweb/ncipc/leadcaus10.html. Accessed May 2012.
13. Karch D, Dahlberg L, Patel N. Surveillance for violent deaths – National Violent Death Reporting System, 16 states, 2007. MMWR. 2010;59(SS04):1–50.
14. Logan J, Smith S. Homicides – United States, 1999–2007. MMWR. 2011;60:67–70.

15. American Association of Suicidology. Suicide in the USA: based on current (2009) statistics. 2012. http://www.suicidology.org/c/document_library/get_file?folderId=262&name=DLFE-532. pdf. Accessed May 2012.
16. Centers for Disease Control and Prevention. Suicide facts at a glance. 2010. http://www.cdc. gov/ViolencePrevention/pdf/Suicide_DataSheet-a.pdf. Accessed May 2012.
17. Centers for Disease Control and Prevention. Suicide prevention. 2012. http://www.cdc.gov/ ViolencePrevention/suicide/index.html. Accessed May 2012.

Conclusions and Recommendations

For 12 of the health conditions studied, South Texas was at a disadvantage compared to the rest of Texas. However, for the remaining 16 health conditions, incidence/mortality rates or prevalence of conditions in South Texas were either lower than or the same as in the rest of Texas (Table 1). For many health conditions, there was a greater occurrence of disease in Hispanics compared to non-Hispanic whites (Table 1). For 11 health conditions, Hispanics in South Texas had higher rates than Hispanics in the rest of Texas (Table 1).

Health Conditions with Lower Rates in South Texas

The following health conditions had lower incidence/mortality rates or prevalence in South Texas than in the rest of Texas:

- HIV/AIDS
- Syphilis
- Gonorrhea
- Breast cancer
- Colorectal cancer
- Prostate cancer
- Lung cancer
- Infant mortality
- Heart disease mortality
- Cerebrovascular disease mortality (stroke)
- Adult current asthma
- Occupational pesticide exposure
- Motor vehicle crash mortality
- Suicide mortality

A.G. Ramirez et al. (eds.), *The South Texas Health Status Review:*
A Health Disparities Roadmap, DOI 10.1007/978-3-319-00233-0, © The Author(s) 2013

Table 1 Comparison of whether South Texas has a higher or lower rate than the rest of Texas or nationwide as well as whether Hispanics have a higher or lower rate than non-Hispanic whites in South Texas for each health condition[a]

Health condition	South Texas as compared with the rest of Texas	South Texas as compared with the Nation	Hispanics in South Texas as compared with non-Hispanic Whites in South Texas	Hispanics in South Texas as compared with Hispanics in the rest of Texas
Tuberculosis	Higher	Higher	Higher	Higher
HIV/AIDS	Lower	[b]	Higher	Lower
Syphilis	Lower	[b]	Higher	Higher
Chlamydia	Higher	[b]	Higher	Higher
Gonorrhea	Lower	[b]	Higher	Higher
Breast cancer	Lower	Lower	Lower	Higher
Cervical cancer	Higher	Higher	Higher	Lower
Colorectal cancer	Lower	Lower		Higher
Prostate cancer	Lower	Lower	Lower	Lower
Lung cancer	Lower	Lower	Lower	
Liver cancer	Higher	Higher	Higher	Higher
Stomach cancer	Higher	Higher	Higher	
Gallbladder cancer	Higher	Higher	Higher	
Leukemia	Higher	Higher	Higher	
Neural tube defects	Higher	[b]	Higher	
Oral clefts		[b]		
Other birth defects	Higher	Higher		
Infant mortality	Lower	[b]	Higher	
Diabetes	Higher	Higher	Higher	Higher
Heart disease mortality	Lower	[b]	Higher	Higher
Cerebrovascular disease mortality	Lower	[b]	Higher	
Obesity (adult)	Higher	Higher	Higher	Higher
Current asthma (adult)	Lower	Lower		
Childhood lead poisoning	Higher	[b]	Higher	
Pesticide exposure	Lower	[b]		
Motor vehicle crash mortality	Lower	[b]		
Homicide mortality			Higher	
Suicide mortality	Lower	Lower	Lower	Higher

[a]Table cells left blank denote similar rates between the two groups being compared
[b]Means that nationwide data were not available to make the comparison between South Texas and the nation

Even though most of the sexually transmitted diseases (HIV/AIDS, syphilis, and gonorrhea) had a lower incidence in South Texas than seen in the rest of Texas, incidence rates of these diseases are higher among Hispanics compared to non-Hispanic whites. The highest rates of these sexually transmitted diseases are seen among African-Americans, who generally reside in the rest of Texas [1, 2].

Historically, the incidence rates of breast, colorectal, prostate, and lung cancer are low in Hispanics compared to other population groups [3]. Not surprisingly, South Texas, with its predominantly Mexican-American population, had lower rates of these cancers than the rest of Texas. Known factors, which may contribute to the lower breast cancer risk in South Texas Hispanics include reproductive factors such as early age at first birth, multiple births, and breast feeding [4]. A diet high in fats, especially animal fats, is a risk factor for breast, colorectal, and prostate cancer [5]. The lower incidence of colorectal and prostate cancer seen in South Texas may be attributable to dietary factors (i.e., a less "western" diet) [6, 7]. It is possible that lower lung cancer incidence rates in South Texas could reflect lower cigarette smoking levels of Hispanics in the past [8].

Overall, lower mortality rates were seen in South Texas for heart disease and cerebrovascular disease. Mortality for these diseases is usually lower among Hispanics than non-Hispanic whites; [9, 10] however, in South Texas, cardiovascular disease mortality rates were higher for Hispanics than for non-Hispanic whites. A high prevalence of obesity and diabetes in South Texas, especially among Hispanics, might contribute to the higher heart disease mortality seen among Hispanics in South Texas.

Because Hispanics in the USA generally have a lower prevalence of asthma than either non-Hispanic whites or African-Americans, the high percentage of Hispanics living in South Texas likely contributed to the lower prevalence of asthma in South Texas compared with the rest of Texas [11]. The incidence of work-related pesticide exposures was also lower in South Texas than in the rest of Texas. This was an unexpected finding, because agriculture is a major industry in South Texas [12]. However, pesticide exposures are underreported throughout the state of Texas, so these estimates might not reflect the true incidence of occupational pesticide exposure in these areas. Mortality due to motor vehicle crashes and suicide was also lower in South Texas than the rest of the state. And notably, the rate of infant mortality was lower in South Texas.

Health Conditions with Higher Rates in South Texas

Several serious conditions had a higher incidence or prevalence in South Texas than in the rest of Texas:

- Tuberculosis
- Chlamydia
- Cervical cancer
- Liver cancer
- Stomach cancer
- Gallbladder cancer
- Child and adolescent leukemia
- Neural tube defects

- Other birth defects (common truncus and pyloric stenosis)
- Adult diabetes
- Adult obesity
- Childhood lead poisoning

Tuberculosis incidence was higher in South Texas than in the rest of Texas or nationwide. The higher incidence of tuberculosis in South Texas is likely due to the higher numbers of foreign-born persons in South Texas, who are more likely to be carriers [13]. Also, South Texas has a larger percentage of individuals with no health insurance than does the rest of Texas, which may contribute to the higher tuberculosis incidence [14].

Several cancers also had a higher incidence in South Texas than in the rest of Texas including cervical cancer, liver cancer, stomach cancer, gallbladder cancer, and child and adolescent leukemia. South Texas women were less likely to have had an up-to-date Pap test than women in the rest of Texas; this lack of screening likely contributes to the higher incidence of primary cervical cancer in South Texas. As well as having a higher incidence in South Texas than the rest of Texas, liver cancer is higher among Hispanics compared to non-Hispanic whites in South Texas and is also higher among Hispanics in South Texas compared to other Hispanics in the rest of the state. Risk factors that may play a role in the increased liver cancer incidence in South Texas include hepatitis B and C infection, aflatoxin-contaminated foods, alcohol consumption or cirrhosis, or genetic factors [15]. Stomach cancer risk is generally associated with lower economic levels and has recently been definitely linked to a chronic bacterial infection with *Helicobacter pylori* [16]. The prevalence of *H. pylori* is high among Hispanics in Texas [17]. The higher prevalence of obesity in South Texas may contribute to the higher incidence of gallbladder cancer, because obesity is a strong risk factor for it [18].

Some birth defects in this study, such as neural tube defects, common truncus, and pyloric stenosis, also had higher prevalences in South Texas than in the rest of Texas. The higher prevalence of these birth defects in South Texas could be associated with inadequate folic acid intake or a higher prevalence of maternal diabetes in South Texas than in the rest of Texas.

The percent of children with elevated blood lead levels was higher in South Texas than in the rest of Texas, but the reason for this is unknown.

One sexually transmitted disease, chlamydia, also had a higher incidence in South Texas than in the rest of Texas. In South Texas, Hispanic individuals and persons living in metropolitan counties had higher incidences of chlamydia than did non-Hispanic whites and non-metropolitan county residents, possibly due to lifestyle factors such as engaging in more risky sexual behaviors.

Lastly, and perhaps most significantly, South Texas had a higher prevalence of both adult obesity and diabetes than did the rest of Texas or nationwide. A significantly higher prevalence of adult diabetes and adult obesity was also observed among Hispanics in South Texas compared to Hispanics in the rest of Texas. These two health conditions go hand in hand; obesity is a risk factor for diabetes. The high prevalence of obesity in South Texas is most likely due to lifestyle behaviors such as inadequate physical activity and poor eating habits [19].

Table 2 Estimates of burden of disease for those health conditions that had a higher incidence or prevalence in South Texas than in the rest of Texas

Health condition	South Texas incidence/ prevalence per 100,000 population	Incidence/prevalence difference between South Texas and the rest of Texas, per 100,000 population
Obesity (adult)	32,700.0	3,600.0
Diabetes (adult)	11,600.0	2,300.0
Childhood lead poisoning	900.0	100.0
Chlamydia	429.4	42.0
Other birth defects	12.6–242.4	5.3–57.1
Neural tube defects	82.3	14.6
Liver cancer	12.2	3.8
Cervical cancer	10.5	1.2
Stomach cancer	8.3	1.6
Tuberculosis	8.2	2.5
Child/adolescent leukemia	5.4	0.8
Gallbladder cancer	1.7	0.6

Many of the health disparities in South Texas may be associated with or exacerbated by the higher percentage of persons with no health insurance in South Texas compared to the rest of Texas. An estimated 30% of the South Texas population has no health insurance, which is a considerable barrier in receiving preventive care or treatment for health conditions [20].

Recommendations

In terms of number of persons affected per 100,000 population, obesity has the greatest impact on South Texans of all the health conditions examined (Table 2). Diabetes has the second-greatest estimated burden of disease in South Texas, followed distantly by childhood lead poisoning. The differences in rates between South Texas and the rest of Texas were also greatest for obesity and diabetes (Table 2). Because these health conditions affect the most people, prevention research efforts in South Texas should focus on obesity and diabetes. Obesity prevention is of special importance, because it increases the risk for diabetes and is also associated with some cancers, cardiovascular disease, and some birth defects. Moreover, because the two modifiable behaviors affecting obesity levels are insufficient physical activity and poor nutrition, these should also be the focus of strategies and intervention research in South Texas.

Insufficient data were available on behavioral risk factor prevalences for South Texas children and adolescents. We recommend that youth behavioral risk factor surveys and studies that focus on the South Texas area be conducted to ascertain behaviors and conditions related to cigarette smoking, alcohol use, asthma, and obesity.

Of epidemiologic interest is the consistently high rate of liver cancer among Hispanics in South Texas. Research on the prevalence and differences with regard to liver cancer risk factors (Hepatitis B and C, aflatoxin exposures, genetic factors) may be informative in this population.

References

1. Centers for Disease Control and Prevention. HIV surveillance report, 2010. vol. 22; 2012. http://www.cdc.gov/hiv/topics/surveillance/resources/reports/. Accessed July 2012.
2. Centers for Disease Control and Prevention. Sexually transmitted disease surveillance 2010. Atlanta: U.S. Department of Health and Human Services, Centers for Disease Control and Prevention; 2011.
3. Ries LAG, Devesa SS. Cancer incidence, mortality, and patient survival in the United States. In: Schottenfeld D, Fraumeni JF, editors. Cancer epidemiology and prevention. 3rd ed. New York: Oxford University Press.; 2006. p. 139–67.
4. Colditz GA, Baer HJ, Tamimi RM. Breast cancer. In: Schottenfeld D, Fraumeni JF, editors. Cancer epidemiology and prevention. 3rd ed. New York: Oxford University Press; 2006. p. 995–1011.
5. Willett WC. Diet and nutrition. In: Schottenfeld D, Fraumeni JF, editors. Cancer epidemiology and prevention. 3rd ed. New York: Oxford University Press; 2006. p. 405–21.
6. Giovannucci E, Wu K. Cancers of the colon and rectum. In: Schottenfeld D, Fraumeni JF, editors. Cancer epidemiology and prevention. 3rd ed. New York: Oxford University Press; 2006. p. 809–29.
7. Platz EA, Giovannucci E. Prostate cancer. In: Schottenfeld D, Fraumeni JF, editors. Cancer epidemiology and prevention. 3rd ed. New York: Oxford University Press; 2006. p. 1128–50.
8. Dube SR, McClave A, James C, Caraballo R, Kaufmann R, Pechacek T. Vital signs: current cigarette smoking among adults aged ≥18 Years – United States, 2009. MMWR. 2010;59:1135–40.
9. Centers for Disease Control and Prevention. Heart disease facts. 2012. http://www.cdc.gov/heartdisease/facts.htm/. Accessed July 2012.
10. Casper ML, Barnett E, Williams Jr GI, Halverson JA, Braham VE, Greenlund KJ. Atlas of stroke mortality: racial, ethnic, and geographic disparities in the United States. Atlanta: Department of Health and Human Services, Centers for Disease Control and Prevention; 2003.
11. American Lung Association. Trends in asthma morbidity and mortality. 2011. http://www.lung.org/finding-cures/our-research/trend-reports/asthma-trend-report.pdf. Accessed July 2012.
12. Texas Comptroller of Public Accounts. Texas in focus: South Texas. 2008. http://www.window.state.tx.us/specialrpt/tif/southtexas/index.html. Accessed July 2012.
13. Miramontes R, Pratt R, Price SF, Jeffries C, Navin TR, Oramasionwu GE. Trends in tuberculosis – United States, 2011. MMWR. 2012;61:181–5.
14. Mayo Clinic Staff. Tuberculosis: risk factors. Mayo Clinic. 2011. http://www.mayoclinic.com/health/tuberculosis/ds00372/dsection=risk-factors. Accessed July 2012.
15. London WT, McGlynn KA. Liver cancer. In: Schottenfeld D, Fraumeni JF, editors. Cancer epidemiology and prevention. 3rd ed. New York: Oxford University Press; 2006. p. 763–86.
16. Shibata A, Parsonnet J. Stomach cancer. In: Schottenfeld D, Fraumeni JF, editors. Cancer epidemiology and prevention. 3rd ed. New York: Oxford University Press; 2006. p. 707–20.
17. Goodman KJ, O'Rourke K, Day RS, Wang C, Redlinger T, Campos A, et al. Helicobacter pylori infection in pregnant women from a U.S.-Mexico border population. J Immigr Health. 2003;5:99–107.
18. American Cancer Society. Gallbladder cancer. 2012. http://www.cancer.org/acs/groups/cid/documents/webcontent/003101-pdf.pdf. Accessed July 2012.
19. Centers for Disease Control and Prevention. Overweight and obesity – causes and consequences. 2012. http://www.cdc.gov/obesity/adult/causes/index.html. Accessed July 2012.
20. Lillie-Blanton M, Hoffman C. The role of health insurance coverage in reducing racial/ethnic disparities in health care. Health Aff. 2005;24:398–408.

Appendix A: Data Sources

Tuberculosis (TB): Statewide TB data is collected by the Infectious Disease Surveillance and Epidemiology Branch of the Infectious Disease Control Unit at the Texas Department of State Health Services (DSHS). TB is a reportable condition in Texas. Statewide tuberculosis surveillance gathers information on individuals with latent TB infection, suspected or active disease, and their contacts; however, only confirmed active disease cases were used in this study's analyses. The Infectious Disease Surveillance and Epidemiology Branch uses passive, active, and sentinel surveillance methods. Crude incidence of TB was calculated for this study.

HIV/AIDS: All confirmed HIV and AIDS cases reported to the State of Texas are contained in the HIV/AIDS Reporting System (HARS) database, which is maintained by the HIV/STD Epidemiology and Surveillance Branch of the Texas Department of State Health Services. When an individual tests positive for HIV, has a detectable viral load, or a CD^4 test with values below 200 or 14 %, the laboratory that runs the test and the health care provider diagnosing the infection are required to report the case to the Texas Department of State Health Services (DSHS). Because HIV infection is a reportable condition, HARS has relatively complete information on persons with HIV in Texas who have tested confidentially for HIV or have sought medical care for their HIV disease. However, the HARS data does not contain information on people living with HIV who are not aware of their infections or persons who know they are infected but have only tested anonymously. As a result, the number of cases provided in DSHS data is an underestimate of all HIV infections in Texas. Active and passive surveillance methods are used to collect HIV/AIDS data. Both confirmed HIV and AIDS cases diagnosed in 2006–2010 were used in this study. HIV and AIDS cases were deduplicated, so that a person diagnosed with both HIV and AIDS during this time period was only counted once. Crude incidence of HIV/AIDS was calculated for this study.

Syphilis, Gonorrhea, and Chlamydia: These sexually transmitted diseases are reportable conditions in Texas and are collected by the HIV/STD Epidemiology and Surveillance Branch of DSHS. The majority of syphilis, chlamydia, and gonorrhea cases are collected using passive surveillance methods such as laboratory and

A.G. Ramirez et al. (eds.), *The South Texas Health Status Review:*
A Health Disparities Roadmap, DOI 10.1007/978-3-319-00233-0, © The Author(s) 2013

provider reporting. However, active surveillance methods are used to investigate early (less than 1 year) syphilis, and approximately 25 % of early syphilis cases in Texas are found by partner elicitation and notification. Gonorrhea and chlamydia cases often have less complete data than syphilis cases, because most chlamydia and gonorrhea cases are discovered through lab reporting, and the sheer volume of these cases makes it hard to follow up on every report that has missing information. Also, because there are 18 local installations of the chlamydia and gonorrhea database rather than one centralized statewide database, there has been little intrastate deduplication of case reports for both chlamydia and gonorrhea. The few duplicate reports that do occur are identified and updated during routine QA processes. Crude incidence of syphilis, gonorrhea, and chlamydia were calculated for this study.

Cancer: The Cancer Epidemiology and Surveillance Branch of the Texas Department of State Health Services collects incident reports of neoplasms occurring among state residents. This information is contained within the Texas Cancer Registry (TCR), a legislatively mandated, statewide, population-based cancer registry. Cancer incidence data are primarily reported to the TCR by more than 500 hospitals, cancer treatment centers, ambulatory surgery centers, and pathology laboratories located throughout the state. Cancer mortality data are extracted from electronic files provided by the Center for Health Statistics at DSHS. These files contain demographic and cause of death information from Texas death certificates for all deaths occurring in Texas.

All cancer incidence and mortality rates were age-adjusted. Age-adjustment is a statistical procedure that eliminates the effects of differences in the age structure between populations and allows direct comparison of incidence and mortality rates between populations. All cancer incidence and mortality rates were age-adjusted to the 2000 US standard million population. Because childhood and adolescent leukemia is so rare, incidence and mortality rates for this type of cancer were expressed per million population at risk rather than per 100,000, which is how the other cancer rates were expressed.

Birth Defects: Data for measuring birth defect occurrence come from two programs at DSHS: the Texas Birth Defects Registry run by the Birth Defects Epidemiology and Surveillance Branch and the birth and fetal death certificate data compiled by the Vital Statistics Unit. Active surveillance is used to gather data for the Texas Birth Defects Registry. Birth defects data are gathered by DSHS staff who routinely visit every Texas hospital, birthing center, or midwife where affected children are born or treated. There, the staff search through log books and hospital discharge lists to look for potential cases. All children with a birth defect covered by British Pediatric Association (BPA) codes 740.000–758.200 have their health data entered into the registry. This process misses children who have birth defects diagnosed after 1 year of age and some pregnancies with birth defects that are terminated in doctors' offices. Aside from those limitations, the data are thought to be very complete. Live birth data are derived from birth certificates, which must by law be completed by the facility delivering the child and sent into DSHS soon after the child's birth. The number of cases of each birth defect is divided by the number of live births and multiplied by 10,000 to yield birth prevalence, expressed as cases per 10,000 live births. By doing this, one can compare birth defect occurrence between different population groups or areas of Texas with different numbers of people. For this study, infants or fetuses with more than one type of birth defect were counted in each relevant category. Crude birth defect prevalence was calculated for this study.

Inadequate Prenatal Care: Prenatal care data was obtained from the Vital Statistics Unit, which is part of the Center for Health Statistics at DSHS. The data are based on information received from Texas birth certificates. Information on whether a mother received prenatal care during the first trimester of pregnancy was used to determine whether she received adequate or inadequate prenatal care during the pregnancy. In this report, the percentage of inadequate prenatal care in each population was defined as the percent of live births whose mothers did not receive prenatal care in the first trimester, out of all live births for which the start month of prenatal care was known.

Mortality Data: In this report, mortality data for all health indicators except cancer were obtained from the Center for Health Statistics at DSHS. Data provided were for Texas residents only. The vital statistics data are based on information received from Texas death certificates. International Statistical Classification of Diseases and Related Health Problems, 10th Revision (ICD-10) codes were used to establish cause of death. Underlying cause of death for mortality data is determined through the use of a computer algorithm developed by the National Center for Health Statistics, called Automated Classification of Medical Entities (ACME). Both underlying and contributing causes of death were taken into account for the diabetes mortality rates shown in this document. For all other mortality indicators except diabetes, only the underlying cause of death was used in the calculation of mortality rates. All mortality measures in this study were age-adjusted to the year 2000 US Standard Population.

Behavioral Risk Factor Data: Data for many health indicators in this document, including those that measured diabetes prevalence, asthma, obesity, no health insurance, physical activity, nutrition, cigarette smoking, alcohol use, and cancer screening behaviors, were collected by the Texas Behavioral Risk Factor Surveillance System (BRFSS). The Texas BRFSS is an annual, statewide telephone survey of Texas adults aged 18 and older that is conducted through a collaborative effort among the federal Centers for Disease Control and Prevention (CDC) and the Texas Department of State Health Services. It is the only state-based surveillance system in Texas that monitors chronic conditions, preventive health practices, and health behaviors. Although some health indicators on the BRFSS survey are part of the core questionnaire and questions are asked about them each year, others are part of the rotating core and asked only every other year. Annual Texas BRFSS data are weighted to adjust for the probabilities of selection (based on the probability of telephone number selection, the number of adults in the household, and the number of residential phone lines) and a poststratification weighting factor that adjusts for sex, age, and white/nonwhite. For this study, BRFSS data from 2007 to 2010 were aggregated and were not reweighted. All prevalence rates and relative risks should be seen as averaged estimates over the data collection years listed in the tables. Calculations of the prevalence estimates, relative risks, and confidence interval limits were performed using SUDAAN (v. 10.0.1), a statistical computing program designed for analyzing data from multistage sample surveys. National data on the behavioral risk factor health indicators listed above were obtained from 2007 to 2010 nationwide BRFSS survey data.

Although the Texas BRFSS provides estimates of many risk factors and health practices that cannot be found in any other data source, there are some limitations to the surveillance system. BRFSS data are based on self-reported information, and, for some indicators, the estimates might be subject to recall bias. BRFSS does not include persons living in nursing homes, prisons, college dormitories, military bases, or other institutions. The BRFSS survey is also currently only conducted by landline telephone and thus excludes those who do not have telephone service or are living in a wireless-only household. Lastly, the BRFSS estimates assume that adults who refuse to do the survey are like those who complete the survey.

BRFSS Health Indicator Prevalence Definitions

- *No Health Insurance*: The proportion of adults who reported to have no health insurance of any kind.
- *Diabetes*: The proportion of adults who had ever been told by a doctor, nurse, or other health professional that they have diabetes. Those who were told that they had diabetes only during pregnancy were considered not to have diabetes.
- *Obesity*: The proportion of adults with a body mass index (BMI) of 30 or greater. BMI was calculated using reported body weight and height information.
- *Inadequate Physical Activity*: The proportion of adults who reported not meeting recommendations for moderate physical activity (at least 30 min, 5 or more days/week) or vigorous physical activity (at least 20 min, 3 or more days/week).
- *Inadequate Fruit and Vegetable Consumption*: The proportion of adults who reported eating fruits and vegetables less than five times per day.
- *Current Smoking*: The proportion of adults who reported having smoked 100 or more cigarettes in their lifetime and who reported still smoking some days or every day.
- *Heavy Alcohol Consumption*: The proportion of adults who reported drinking, on average, more than two drinks per day (for men) or more than one drink per day (for women) in the past 30 days.
- *Binge Drinking*: The proportion of adults who reported drinking five or more drinks for men, or four or more drinks for women, on one or more occasions in the past 30 days.
- *Current Asthma*: The proportion of adults who reported having ever been diagnosed with asthma by a doctor, nurse, or other health professional, and who still have asthma symptoms.

- *No Mammogram*: The proportion of adult females aged 40 and older who reported not having a mammogram within the past 2 years.
- *No Pap Test*: The proportion of adult females with an intact uterine cervix who reported not having a Pap test within the past 3 years.
- *No PSA Test*: The proportion of adult males aged 40 and older who reported not having a PSA test within the past 2 years.
- *No Digital Rectal Exam (DRE)*: The proportion of adult males aged 40 and older who reported not having a DRE within the past 5 years.
- *No Fetal Occult Blood Test (FOBT)*: The proportion of adults aged 50 and older who reported not having a FOBT within the past 2 years.
- *No Sigmoidoscopy/Colonoscopy*: The proportion of adults aged 50 and older who reported never having a sigmoidoscopy or colonoscopy test.

Pregnancy Risk Assessment Monitoring System Data: In this report, data on pregnancy intention, prepregnancy overweight and obesity, and prepregnancy health insurance coverage were obtained from the Texas Pregnancy Risk Assessment Monitoring System (PRAMS). In partnership with the Centers for Disease Control and Prevention (CDC) and the Texas Department of State Health Services (DSHS), Texas PRAMS is a population-based survey that monitors maternal attitudes and behaviors before, during, and after pregnancy. The PRAMS study population includes all women with a live birth[1] delivering in Texas in a given year. A monthly stratified sample of mothers is selected from the birth file based on race/ethnicity and infant birth weight. Sampled women are recruited to participate in PRAMS through two modes of data collection—mail and telephone. Women are first sent a survey through the mail when their infants are approximately 60–90 days old; there are multiple attempts to get a completed mailed survey. If they do not complete and return the survey through the mail, they are advanced into the telephone phase of data collection.

To make the data representative of all live births in Texas, the CDC calculates an analysis weight for each respondent. The analysis weight can be interpreted as the number of women in the population that each individual respondent represents. For this report, PRAMS data from the 2004 to 2009 birth years were aggregated. SAS software version 9.2 was used for all analyses, and the complex sampling scheme of PRAMS was accounted for in the analyses.

It is important to understand the limitations of PRAMS data. These limitations may contribute to unreliable estimates, as well as variations in prevalence when comparing PRAMS to other data sources such as birth certificate data. One limitation inherent to self-reported survey data is the potential for recall bias and/or misinterpretation of questions. Additionally, the Texas PRAMS data are weighted to the

---

[1] Adoptive mothers are excluded from the sample. Additionally, the sampling procedures include coding that randomly selects only one infant from a multiple gestation. Multiple births of four or more are excluded.

state population; the South Texas PRAMS data presented in this report were not reweighted. Although sample bias assessment and response pattern comparison were conducted and bias was found to be minimal, if the data were to be reweighted in the future, the estimates could vary from those provided here. Lastly, the CDC sets response rate threshold guidelines for minimal nonresponse bias. Texas met this response rate threshold (65 %) in 2009 but fell short of the minimum response rate for years 2004 to 2008. For more details about PRAMS, please visit http://www.dshs.state.tx.us/mch/default.shtm#PRAMS2 or http://www.cdc.gov/prams/.

PRAMS Health Indicator Prevalence Definitions

- Unintended pregnancy: The estimated percent of respondents who reported that *just before* they got pregnant, they felt that they "wanted to be pregnant later" or that they "didn't want to be pregnant then or at any time in the future."
- Prepregnancy obesity: The estimated percent of respondents with a BMI of 30 or higher.
- Prepregnancy overweight: The estimated percent of respondents with a BMI between 25 and 29.9.
- No health insurance before pregnancy: The estimated percent of respondents who reported that they did not have health insurance *just before* pregnancy or the *month before* pregnancy.

Childhood Lead Poisoning: Statewide blood/lead testing results for children aged 0–14 are collected by the Childhood Lead Poisoning Prevention Program (CLPPP) of the Texas Department of State Health Services. Reporting data on Texas children who are tested for lead, along with associated test-related and patient demographic information, is required from all health care providers and laboratories. For the purposes of this analysis, a child was considered to have an elevated blood lead level if ≥ 10 µg/dL of lead was found in the blood through one or more blood tests during the study timeframe (2006–2010). Most childhood lead poisoning surveillance data are not collected to calculate prevalence or incidence of lead poisoning, because lead screening data are not collected by a random or a complete census, screening rates are low, and provider screening practices may change over time. Typically childhood morbidity data is expressed as a percentage of elevated children among those tested, as was done in this study.

Pesticide Exposure: Pesticide exposure data are collected by the Pesticide Exposure Surveillance in Texas (PEST) Program of DSHS. PEST receives the majority of its data from the Texas Poison Center Network (TPCN). Physicians, laboratory directors, and health professionals are also required to report acute occupational pesticide poisoning. The program also obtains case reports from other state agencies and departments such as the Texas Department of Agriculture (including the Texas Structural Pest Control Service) and the Texas Department of Insurance Division of Workers' Compensation. Even though only occupational pesticide exposure is required to be reported to the state, the PEST program does obtain counts of both occupational and nonoccupational pesticide exposure calls received by the Texas Poison Center Network. However, because reporting is not required for nonoccupational pesticide exposure cases, these numbers are likely underreported. This report only includes data on occupational pesticide exposures. Both active and passive surveillance methods are used to gather pesticide exposure data. PEST staff begin the surveillance process within 24 h of receiving a report, attempting to locate the individual for an interview and requesting related medical records. Occasionally, medical records provide the only source of data for a case; most case data, however, is compiled from the original report, the individual interview, and the case medical records. Only confirmed cases were used in this report's incidence analyses; these are cases that meet the Sentinel Event Notification System for Occupational Risk (SENSOR) criteria of a confirmed case. To determine a confirmed case, reports must specify the pesticide, health effects, and a consistent association between health effects and the known toxicology of the pesticide. Based on the level that case data meet the confirmed criteria, confirmed cases are further subdivided into four categories: definite, probable, possible, and suspicious. All of these categories were included in this report's pesticide exposure analyses. Crude incidence of pesticide exposure was calculated for this report.

Denominator Data: The Texas population estimates and projections used as denominator data to help generate the incidence, prevalence, and mortality rates in this report were provided by the Population Estimates and Projections Program of the Texas State Data Center. Population estimates were used for the years 2004–2009, and population projections published in 2008 were used for 2010 population data.

Appendix B: Data Analysis Methods

For each health indicator, overall incidence/mortality rates or prevalence were obtained both for the 38-county South Texas area and the rest of Texas. Crude incidence or prevalence estimates were used for some health indicators, while age-adjusted estimates were used for others (e.g., all mortality data and cancer data). Race/ethnicity-stratified rates were also obtained for South Texas and the rest of Texas. For some health indicators (BRFSS indicators, PRAMS indicators, and birth defects), rates for South Texas and the rest of Texas were compared by calculating a rate ratio (South Texas rate/rest of Texas rate). A 95 % confidence interval (CI) was calculated for the rate ratio and was used to determine if the South Texas estimate was statistically significantly different from the rest of Texas estimate (we stated that the incidence/mortality rate or prevalence was different in South Texas than in the rest of Texas if the rate ratio's 95 % confidence interval did not include 1.0). For all other health indicators, 95 % CIs were calculated around estimates for South Texas and the rest of Texas. If these 95 % CIs did not overlap, we stated that there was a significant difference in incidence, mortality, or prevalence between South Texas and the rest of Texas.

For the South Texas area, age- and sex- stratified rates were also calculated for each health indicator, as well as separate rates for metropolitan and nonmetropolitan counties and for Bexar County, Webb County, and the Lower Rio Grande Valley region, if the number of cases permitted. For all incidence/mortality rates or prevalence estimates, a 95 % confidence interval was calculated. This confidence interval was used to determine whether or not different groups within South Texas (e.g., male vs. female) had statistically significantly different rates. If the groups' 95 % CIs did not overlap, we stated that there was a difference in incidence, prevalence, or mortality between the groups.

A.G. Ramirez et al. (eds.), *The South Texas Health Status Review:* *A Health Disparities Roadmap*, DOI 10.1007/978-3-319-00233-0, © The Author(s) 2013

Appendix C: South Texas County Demographics, 2010

County name	Estimated population	Percent Hispanic	Percent of persons living below poverty level
Atascosa County	45,883	63.7	20.4
Bandera County	21,266	14.6	16.5
Bee County	34,105	57.4	27.3
Bexar County	1,636,642	59.0	17.0
Brooks County	7,866	91.1	33.0
Cameron County	417,404	87.2	35.8
Comal County	121,020	22.7	11.9
Dimmit County	9,761	84.1	31.0
Duval County	12,041	86.7	26.9
Edwards County	2,213	49.2	25.3
Frio County	17,956	75.8	35.3
Gillespie County	25,873	17.6	12.1
Guadalupe County	128,975	39.3	11.4
Hidalgo County	793,137	91.5	33.4
Jim Hogg County	5,506	89.7	24.8
Jim Wells County	42,455	77.8	21.6
Karnes County	16,838	50.2	26.3
Kendall County	35,351	19.4	10.0
Kenedy County	470	79.6	12.5
Kerr County	46,829	24.2	15.6
Kinney County	3,449	57.0	24.7
Kleberg County	31,990	65.9	24.6
La Salle County	6,029	77.4	34.4
Live Oak County	12,409	42.5	18.6
McMullen County	878	34.5	11.9
Maverick County	55,221	95.4	39.9
Medina County	45,657	49.3	17.5
Nueces County	323,890	63.3	20.0
Real County	3,351	22.6	24.1
San Patricio County	70,895	53.7	21.1
Starr County	67,382	97.9	39.2

A.G. Ramirez et al. (eds.), *The South Texas Health Status Review:*
A Health Disparities Roadmap, DOI 10.1007/978-3-319-00233-0, © The Author(s) 2013

County name	Estimated population	Percent Hispanic	Percent of persons living below poverty level
Uvalde County	27,857	70.9	26.4
Val Verde County	50,067	78.2	26.8
Webb County	257,590	95.2	31.5
Willacy County	22,035	87.9	36.9
Wilson County	45,517	39.3	12.1
Zapata County	15,266	89.8	32.3
Zavala County	12,844	92.2	36.9

Source: Texas Health Data (http://soupfin.tdh.state.tx.us/people.htm); 2010 projection data were used. 2010 poverty estimates obtained from the US Census Bureau (http://www.census.gov//did/www/saipe/index.html)

Index

A.G. Ramirez et al. (eds.), *The South Texas Health Status Review:*
A Health Disparities Roadmap, DOI 10.1007/978-3-319-00233-0, © The Author(s) 2013